Beyond
APHASIA

Titles in the **Speechmark Editions** series:

Beyond APHASIA

Therapies for Living with
Communication Disability

Carole Pound, Susie Parr,
Jayne Lindsay & Celia Woolf

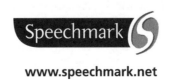

Speechmark

www.speechmark.net

Carole Pound is a speech & language therapist with a specialist interest in neurorehabilitation. Since 1994 she has been Director of the City Dysphasic Group (Aphasia Centre, London), a therapy and support centre for people with long-term aphasia, based at City University. Current clinical and research interests include developing and evaluating living with aphasia therapies, describing, implementing and integrating impairment and non-impairment therapies, training volunteers and relatives as conversation partners and working with relatives and caregivers.

Susie Parr has worked as a speech & language therapist in Ireland, Liverpool and Bristol. She is currently Research Fellow at the Department of Clinical Communication Studies, City University. She has carried out research into aphasia and literacy, the social consequences of aphasia and the experience of language impairment.

Jayne Lindsay joined the staff of the City Dysphasic Group in 1995. Previously she worked extensively with people with communication and swallowing problems in all stages of the rehabilitative process, and still lectures on all aspects of dysphagia and dysarthria. Her current clinical and research interests include the application of Conversation Analysis to aphasic talk, and the potential for non-speech methods of communication to reveal the competence of people with severe aphasia.

Celia Woolf is a speech & language therapist with a specialist interest in community-based therapy for adults. After completing the Advanced Clinical Studies in Aphasia, she joined the team at the City Dysphasic Group in 1995. Her clinical and research interests include evaluating group therapy, goal setting, stress management and access based therapies. She is currently embarking on PhD studies into auditory processing impairments in aphasia at University College London.

Published by
Speechmark Publishing Ltd, 70 Alston Drive, Bradwell Abbey,
Milton Keynes MK13 9HG, UK
www.speechmark.net

© Carole Pound, Susie Parr, Jayne Lindsay & Celia Woolf, 2000

First published 2000
Reprinted 2001, 2002, 2004, 2006, 2008

002-3842/Printed in the United Kingdom/1010

British Library Cataloguing in Publication Data

Pound, Carole
    Beyond aphasia: therapies for living with communication disability – (Speechmark editions)
    1. Aphasia – Treatment
    I. Pound, Carole
    616.8'552'06

ISBN: 978 0 86388 347 7

Contents

Figures

Tables

Foreword

THIS IMPORTANT VOLUME documents both the practical and philosophical experience and thinking of an outstanding team of aphasiologists at the aphasia centre affiliated with the City University in London. It is aptly titled *Beyond Aphasia*. Indeed, by addressing the socially disabling consequences of aphasia, the authors have made a case for the political and social challenge to remove the barriers of bias and inaccessibility that face people with aphasia. Following a social disability model embedded in a thoughtful philosophy which speaks for the re-establishment of personal and collective identity as necessary for living with aphasia, a design for aphasia management is presented. The work focuses on the disabling effects of aphasia whether objectively observed, inferred or subjectively experienced by the individual. In so doing it moves away from the medical tradition of focusing on impairment to the realm of individual, idiosyncratic experience. This view of aphasia as a social disability casts the problem in a cultural and ethnological context.

By emphasising the invisibility of aphasia and its inevitable negative effect on the individual's ability to participate in a world of speakers, the authors define the context in which persons with aphasia can best be managed. Acknowledging the uniqueness and complexity of the individual and his/her communication universe is as fundamental in the design of a complete approach to aphasia management, they succeed in embracing the perspectives of different disciplines and, remarkably, bringing them together into a comprehensive and cohesive whole. The detailed descriptive analysis of the activities which comprise the core of the aphasia centre programme offers powerful support for the person with aphasia as someone with specific and generally unmet needs. While patient autonomy, empowerment, advocacy and choice are essential goals of the work they do not deny the importance of improving communication through the development of compensatory strategies, training conversation partners and other venues.

In addition to its significance as an important philosophical statement this volume is a superb resource for creatively analysed and constructed materials that address the psychosocial consequences of aphasia. The integration of a broad spectrum of current thought to the amelioration of the devastating effects of chronic aphasia into a larger rehabilitation scheme, enhanced by the authors' creative thinking represents a major contribution to our knowledge.

Martha Taylor Sarno, MA MDhc
Professor, Department of Rehabilitation Medicine
New York University School of Medicine
Director, Speech-Language Pathology Department

Preface

THIS BOOK DESCRIBES AN APPROACH to therapy and support for people who live with long-term communication disability. This approach underpins the work of the aphasia centre attached to City University, London, which has attracted national and international interest because of its innovative practice. The centre started life in the 1970s as the Blackfriars Group, providing therapy for people with aphasia and training for speech and language therapy students. In 1984, it was incorporated into the university and is currently part of the Department of Language and Communication Science, which offers courses leading to professional qualifications in speech and language therapy. The centre provides clinical experience and supervision for the undergraduate and postgraduate students who largely comprise its workforce. However, it has independent status and its work is funded largely through charitable donations.

The aphasia centre has recently attracted major funding from the Dunhill Medical Trust which will support the development, over a period of five years, of a national network of centres for people with communication disabilities. This initiative will be known as the Connect Network.

At present, people come to the aphasia centre from all parts of London and its neighbouring counties. The service offered by the centre is integrated with the speech and language therapy services offered by local and neighbouring NHS trusts. Typically, clients attend for two full days weekly and are offered a flexible package of group and individual work, with termly review. Thirty-four weeks of therapy are offered each year (to accord with the university terms). Out of term time, we offer training courses designed to support and develop the expertise of those who are concerned with aphasia, including volunteers, family members and professionals. Work at the centre is informed by research into aphasia carried out within the university department and elsewhere. We have established links within the international research community, and with similar centres in the USA and Canada.

Over the past five years, the aphasia centre has drawn upon a range of therapeutic traditions but has also been much influenced by ideas from other disciplines, particularly disability theory. The approach which is evolving at the centre is unusual in offering an integrated approach to therapy, at once seeking to address language impairment but also focusing upon the struggles which people who are living with long-term communication disability experience. This integrated approach and the innovative therapies that are evolving have attracted interest on a national and international scale.

Beyond Aphasia has been conceived as a response to the numerous requests which we receive for information about the philosophy and practice of the aphasia centre. It seeks to make explicit the principles underpinning the work of the centre, and to outline the practicalities and pitfalls of implementing the ideas which have developed. The focus of the book falls upon therapies for living with communication disabilities, as these are relatively new and unexplored. Impairment-focused therapies are well described elsewhere (for example, Byng *et al*, 1999). Their contribution to the advancement of aphasia therapy is widely acknowledged. For this reason they are given relatively little priority within this text.

In this book, we describe some of the therapeutic methods and interventions which are being developed at the aphasia centre. In Chapter 1, we describe the theoretical background to the work of the centre, and give an overview of the range of interventions offered. Chapter 2 outlines the principles of groupwork and shared goal planning which underpin our approach. Chapter 3 addresses the development and maintenance of communication skills. It describes therapies which focus on developing the skills both of the person with aphasia and those within surrounding social networks and communities. In Chapter 4, we consider the nature of the disabling barriers that are faced by the person with aphasia, and outline some therapies which make a start on dismantling them. We address the complex issue of identity in Chapter 5, and describe ways in which therapeutic interventions can support the development and maintenance of the personal, social and collective identities of people with aphasia. In the final chapter, we chart the various courses through therapy taken by different clients, together with our thoughts on the point and process of leaving therapy, evaluating change and the dilemmas raised by an integrated approach. We also look at how the approaches to therapy that we use at the aphasia centre might be adapted for use in different environments – for example, in a hospital setting.

It is hoped that *Beyond Aphasia* will be useful to practitioners and therapists working in different settings, to students of speech and language therapy and psychology, to disability theorists, to those working with caregivers and volunteers, and to all those concerned with the nature of long-term language disability and its impact on individuals, families and communities. We hope that the book will extend understanding of communication disability, and contribute to the theory and practice of aphasia therapy.

Carole Pound
Susie Parr
Jayne Lindsay
Celia Woolf

London, 2000

Acknowledgements

THE IDEAS AND ACTIVITIES IN THIS BOOK are the result of a five-year period of collaboration. There are many people who have contributed generously to this process. First and foremost, we thank the people with aphasia, their relatives and all the student keyworkers at City University who have generated, challenged and participated in the activities we present here.

We thank also our colleagues at City University and in the profession who have supported and contributed to the work discussed here. In particular, we are grateful to Liz Clark, Hetty Lynn, Sue Whitehead, Deborah Morgan, Winifred Peacock, Chris Ireland, Sue Boazman, Harry Clarke and John Wharton who contribute in many different ways to the work of the centre; to Jane Marshall, Jo Robson, Karen Bunning, Nicola Grove for their insights on aphasia, advocacy and literature; to Liz Syed for her help with the illustrations; and to Tom Penman, Cathy Sparkes and Anne Whateley for their thoughts on applying these practices to other settings. We are particularly grateful to Sally Byng for her vision in developing the content, direction and boundaries of aphasia therapy in the United Kingdom. Our work has also drawn on the ideas and practice of our colleagues overseas. We would especially like to thank Rozanne Barrow, Bronwyn Davidson, Judy Duchan, Roberta Elman, Aura Kagan, Guylaine Le Dorze, Jon Lyon, Martha Taylor Sarno and Nina Simmons-Mackie who, with their respective colleagues, have fed the work of the centre with new ideas and initiatives.

ACKNOWLEDGEMENTS

Finally, as a charitably funded centre, we thank all those trusts, companies and individuals who have generously sponsored the work of the centre and enabled the development and dissemination of the ideas presented in this text.

CHAPTER 1

Developing Therapies for Living with Communication Disability

THE STARTING POINT for the work of the aphasia centre is the experience of living with aphasia. People who have aphasia describe the dramatic and often traumatic nature of its onset, the sense of bewilderment and fear which loss of language engenders, its impact on their lives, families and work, their day-to-day struggles with interaction, conversation and communication, and the profound and often long-term adjustments which must be made. The multi-faceted nature of aphasia demands a flexible, integrated approach to therapy and support.

The service which is evolving at the aphasia centre draws upon a number of different influences, both within aphasiology and beyond, and aims to achieve balance and integration in what is offered to clients. In this chapter, we describe some of these formative influences, focusing particularly on those which come from outside the domain of traditional aphasiology.

Influences within aphasiology

At the aphasia centre, clients are offered a range of options for therapy that draw upon diverse sources and traditions. Some of these are rooted in well established, theoretically based therapeutic approaches to language impairment. For example, in the 1980s, the therapy programmes offered at the centre were profoundly influenced by the rapid developments within cognitive neuropsychology. Cognitive neuropsychologically based interventions continue to play a major role in contemporary aphasia therapy, and to grow in sophistication. They create opportunities for precise specification of language processing breakdowns and the development of targeted, rational interventions (Byng *et al*, 1990; Thompson, 1998).

Clients attending the aphasia centre have the opportunity to analyse and work on their language impairment using these principles – often a prerequisite to disability-focused therapy. Because cognitive neuropsychological methods are extremely well documented, they do not form the main focus of this book. However, the flexible combination of approaches forms a recurring theme throughout the text and in each chapter the integration of methods is discussed.

Other aphasiological traditions that have influenced the work of the centre include Holland's work on functional communication (Holland, 1982), which is concerned with re-establishing the aphasic person's use of effective communication in everyday contexts, and Total Communication, which focuses upon encouraging multi-modality interactions (Lawson & Fawcus, 1999).

We try to be alert to new theoretical and clinical developments within established therapeutic traditions and to feed these into the work of the centre. For example, the practice of aphasia therapy has been influenced in the 1990s by new approaches to the modification of the language environment that surrounds the person with aphasia. Jon Lyon's work on the use of drawing to enhance communication (Lyon, 1995) has extended the scope both of the functional approach and of Total Communication. Dr Lyon visited the centre in 1996 and worked with some of the clients. A research project on communicative drawing was being carried out at the centre at the time. This explored the potential of training people with severe aphasia to make use of drawing skills in backing up their communication (Sacchett *et al*, 1999).

Another major influence on aphasia therapy in the 1990s has been the work on training conversation partners developed at the Pat Arato Aphasia Centre, Toronto (Kagan, 1998). Strong links have been formed between the centres in London and Toronto. Working to extend and develop the skills of conversation partners, whether friends, family members, volunteers, students or professionals, has subsequently become a major focus of our work. Interventions that aim to reconnect people who have aphasia with their communities, and to support their caregivers (Lyon *et al*, 1997) have also influenced the practice of the centre. The philosophical underpinnings of what might be called a 'systemic' approach (that is, one which pays attention to the social networks of which the person with aphasia is a part, as well as to the language impairment itself) have been strengthened by the growth of literature concerning the 'co-construction' of aphasia:

> As an injury, aphasia does reside in the skull. However, as a form of life, a way of being and acting in the world in concert with others, its proper locus is an endogenous, distributed, multi-party system. (Goodwin, 1995, p31)

Of course, aphasiologists like Martha Taylor Sarno have long been concerned not just with the functional impact of aphasia but with the psychosocial effects upon the individuals who have it and the communities of which they are a part. Describing aphasia as a 'social problem', Sarno (1997) urges that increased attention be paid to its social ramifications. Her perspective encapsulates the therapies for living with aphasia which we are trying to develop at the centre:

> National and regional aphasia associations must be strengthened, supported and encouraged to develop networks of aphasia advocacy groups in a cross-section of communities. In this regard we need to reach out to new aphasic patients, their caregivers, primary care physicians and health personnel at the community level and provide broad-based public education which informs and guides them to the best resources for support, acceptance, social interaction and community integration. (Sarno, 1997, pp676–7)

3

Influences beyond aphasiology: the impact of social model theory

While the influences described in the last section largely emerge from traditions within aphasiology, developments within disability theory have also had a major impact on the philosophy and practice of the centre. Readers with an aphasiological background may not be familiar with these concepts, and for this reason we are devoting the rest of this chapter to describing them in some detail.

Thinkers within the disability movement have reconceptualised disability in a way that profoundly challenges the assumptions and traditions of the rehabilitation culture and raises important questions for all those offering therapeutic services to people with aphasia. These concern four central issues:

- Alternative conceptualisations or models of disability
- The experience of disabled people
- Issues of empowerment and emancipation
- The relationship between impairment and disability.

In the following sections of this chapter we will outline these issues, then give an overview of how they influence the work of the centre.

Alternative models of disability

Disability theorists have shown that disability can be conceptualised in a number of different ways, some of which have more cultural power than others. Over the past decade, a number of different 'models' of disability have been described, each offering different constructions of disability. Reflection on these different models promotes understanding that disability is as much a cultural process as a biomedical state. Three contrasting models of disability are the medical model, the philanthropic model and the social model.

Medical model of disability

This model of disability underpins traditional approaches to the rehabilitation of disabled people and, as such, will be familiar to every aphasia therapist. Essentially, the medical model of disability focuses upon the functional inabilities and limitations of the disabled individual.

Disability is seen as an inevitable corollary of impairment. Rehabilitation traditionally takes place within a medical context and culture, and is imbued with medical language and concepts. Medical model interventions aim to reduce the individual's impairment and restore maximum function and independence. The medical model was encapsulated in the International Classification of Impairments, Disabilities and Handicaps developed by the World Health Organisation in 1980:

Impairment Any loss or abnormality of psychological, physiological or anatomical structure or function.

Disability Any restriction or lack of ability to perform an activity as a result of impairment, in a manner, or within the range which is considered normal for a human being.

Handicap A disadvantage for a given individual, resulting from an impairment or a disability, that limits or prevents the fulfilment of a role which is normal for that individual (depending on such factors as age, sex and social or cultural factors).

In 1997, the World Health Organisation updated the 1980 model, replacing the terms 'disability' with 'activities' and 'handicap' with 'participation'.

The philanthropic model of disability
The philanthropic model of disability informs much of the work undertaken on behalf of disabled people by voluntary and charitable organisations. It has been most critically and comprehensively described in an analysis of representations of disabled people in charity advertising (Hevey, 1992). Through the use of particular forms of visual and verbal imagery, disabled people have been variously represented in charity advertisements as tragic, brave objects of pity, or as heroically overcoming their impairments. Either way, it is suggested that they are dependent upon charitable support, and grateful for it.

The philanthropic model has a profound influence upon media accounts of disability, as a glance through any tabloid or local newspaper will confirm. However, alternative images of disabled people are starting to emerge. For example, recent fashion initiatives display, celebrate and play upon motor and sensory impairments and effectively reconfigure disabled people as sexualised, image-conscious consumers (as described in a feature in the September 1998 issue of *Dazed and Confused*).

Disability theorists are starting to deconstruct the pity and fear with which disabled people have traditionally been regarded, and to explore these stigmatising reactions within the context of cultural and economic factors. Analysis of cultural stigma explores, among other things, the relationship between economic productivity and able-bodiment. This relationship was transformed with industrialisation – a process that rendered people with physical impairments effectively non-productive and economically worthless (Barnes, 1996). A concept such as this seems relevant to aphasia as, in the late 1990s, fast, effective, multi-channel communication has become an essential feature and component of productivity. 'Communication skills' feature in every work appraisal and school report. This may offer some explanation for the fact that people with aphasia, whose communication skills are compromised, describe a sense of being stigmatised and culturally sanctioned.

The social model of disability

The social model of disability emerged within British disability theory and offers an alternative construction to dominant medical and philanthropic philosophies. The social model challenges the medical model by reconfiguring disability in terms of social oppression and by questioning the function and nature of rehabilitation itself. According to this model, disability does not inevitably stem from the functional limitations of impaired individuals, but from the failure of the social and physical environment to take account of their needs. It is 'a political issue, a matter of civil rights, not medical needs' (Abberley, 1991, p174). While the social model definition of impairment remains largely the same, the concept of 'handicap' disappears, and disability is reconceptualised:

Disability is the loss or limitation of opportunities that prevents people who have impairments from taking part in the normal life of the community on an equal level with others due to physical and social barriers. (Finkelstein & French, 1993, p28)

Like other models of disability, the social model is intrinsically complex and constantly evolving. It draws on many influences, particularly anti-sexist and anti-racist movements. However, it can be fairly succinctly described in terms of two key concepts: disabling barriers and the disabled identity.

Disabling barriers

According to the social model, people are disabled, not by their own inabilities but by the socially constructed barriers which spring up around them. These can take a variety of forms:

> All disabled people experience disability as a social restriction, whether these restrictions occur as a consequence of inaccessible built environments, questionable notions of intelligence and social competence, the inability of the general public to use sign-language, the lack of reading material in Braille, or hostile public attitudes to people with non-visible disabilities. (Oliver, 1996, p33)

Oliver's description indicates the range and diversity of disabling barriers. *Environmental* barriers are perhaps most obvious when the experience of people who have motor or sensory impairments is considered. People are disabled not by an inability to walk or see, but by narrow doorways, stairs, lack of ramps and lifts, inaccessible public transport and so on. *Structural* barriers arise when resources, services and opportunities are not available, appropriate or accessible. *Informational* barriers arise when information is unavailable, irrelevant or incomprehensible. *Attitudinal* barriers are evident when people who have impairments encounter hostility and discrimination.

A recent qualitative study of the experience of people with aphasia, carried out in City University, identified some of the numerous disabling barriers facing people who have acquired language impairment (Parr *et al*, 1997). *Environmental* barriers include background noise, which can make it more difficult for the person with aphasia to process what is being said. In addition, the person with aphasia operates not just within a physical environment, but within a language environment. The spoken and written language which surrounds the person with aphasia is effectively disabling if it is too fast, too complex or too oblique.

Structural barriers spring up when the person with aphasia finds it difficult to access rights, resources, opportunities or services – by no means an uncommon experience for the respondents in the study. People with aphasia, for example, may find it difficult to understand their eligibility for benefits and to negotiate the process of claiming them. This, in part, is due to difficulty finding and accessing information which is often incomprehensible to people with language impairment. This constitutes another barrier. In addition, people with aphasia face *attitudinal* barriers in the form of other people's incomprehension, pity, fear and even hostility.

Disability and identity
The notion of identity is also central to the social model philosophy. In part, the notion of identity concerns the self-image and self-understanding of disabled people and the endeavour to celebrate difference in the face of negative, pitying representations of impairment. This is seen as:

> a challenge to dominant social perceptions of disability as a personal tragedy and the affirmation of positive images of disability through development of a politics of personal identity. (Oliver, 1996, p89)

However, disability theorists have also addressed the complex issue of social identity, reflecting upon disabled people's membership of, or exclusion from, groups, communities and cultures (Corker, 1996). The rise of disabled people as a cohesive political force also manifests the growth of what has been called a 'collective identity'.

The disabled person's development of strong personal, social and collective identity is by no means a straightforward or inevitable process. Many disabled people, including some with aphasia, have no desire to see their situation in political terms. Aphasia is a particularly challenging impairment, because it is essentially invisible. People who have hidden impairments may wish to keep them hidden. People with aphasia have to make decisions about whether or not to reveal it and this can influence whether or not they join with others similarly affected. In addition, many disabled people understand and represent their own experience in the terms of powerful, culturally dominant models of disability. Acquired impairments such as aphasia may lead to many personal and social identity entanglements, as the disabled person struggles to reconcile the past with the new situation. Sophisticated methods of analysing narrative and discourse (that is, the ways in which people talk and write about disability) afford some insight into how disabled people form, develop and maintain their identities, and how they can be disrupted (Corker & French, 1999).

In order to clarify the conceptual differences between the social model of disability and other culturally dominant models, Oliver (1996) collapsed the medical and philanthropic constructions into one 'individual' model of disability. The distinctions he points out between the principles underpinning the two models show clearly how a social model definition of disability places the locus of responsibility for disability upon society, rather than upon the individual (*see* Table 1.1).

Table 1.1 *A comparison of individual and social models of disability*

Individual model	Social model
Personal tragedy	Social oppression
Personal problem	Social problem
Individual treatment	Social action
Medicalisation	Self-help
Professional dominance	Individual and collective responsibility
Expertise	Experience
Adjustment	Affirmation
Individual identity	Collective identity
Prejudice	Discrimination
Behaviour	Attitudes
Care	Rights
Control	Choice
Policy	Politics
Individual adaptation	Social change

Source: (Oliver, 1996).

Clearly, the social model of disability levels a major challenge at those who work within medical and philanthropic institutions and cultures. Some disability theorists have been particularly harsh in their critique of the professions concerned with the rehabilitation of disabled people. Therapists, doctors, rehabilitation personnel and researchers are described as having promoted the dependency of disabled people in order to maintain their own work structures and lifestyles (Oliver, 1996). The rehabilitation 'industry' is seen to be concerned only with 'normalising' impairment, and to disregard the numerous extraneous political, economic and social factors that constitute the lived experience of disability.

According to this argument, the professional gaze is focused upon isolated components of impairment related to specific expertise. Thus, in their dealings with a person who has had a stroke, physiotherapists may concentrate upon gait and balance, an occupational therapist upon perception, getting to the toilet, and safety, a speech and language therapist upon swallowing, comprehension and use of language, a doctor upon blood pressure and clotting rates and so on:

> The reality, of course, is that disabled people's lives cannot be divided up in this way to suit professional activity and, increasingly, disabled people, individually and collectively, are coming to reject the prescriptions of the normalising society and the whole range of professional activities which attempt to reinforce it. (Oliver, 1996, p37)

In recent years, some attention has been paid to social model thinking within aphasiology. In particular, Jordan and Kaiser (1996) explored the implications of social model philosophy for the provision of therapy services, and Jordan (1998) has reiterated the challenge posed to therapists:

> The individual and social models of disability offer competing ideologies, not just for aphasia therapy but for speech and language therapy more generally, for other therapies, and, indeed, for all work with disabled people. As I have shown, the values of the social model are beginning to be adopted internationally, and there is thus a strong case for the therapy professions (and everyone else) to embrace them. (Jordan, 1998, p479)

The experience of disabled people

One of the many criticisms levelled at rehabilitation professionals by social model thinkers is that they base their interventions upon non-disabled assumptions about what it must be like to experience impairment. These effectively undermine the subjective experience of disabled people. From a social model perspective, the subjective experience of disabled people needs to be explored and offers significant insights into the nature of disability: the personal story has political potential.

This idea has influenced a number of initiatives within disability theory and research. Accounts of the personal experience of impairment are now forming the basis for in-depth theoretical analysis (Corker and French, 1999). Increasingly, social research into disability is endeavouring to explore the subjective experience of impairment (for example, Morris, 1998; Goldsmith, 1996).

The subjective experience of aphasia

The subjective experience of people with language impairments has been relatively little explored. Reasons for the exclusion of people who are 'inarticulate' from social research seem complex and are not yet fully understood (Booth, 1996). Certainly, in terms of aphasia, personal stories have largely been used as material for 'expert' commentary, although this is now starting to change (Boazman, 1999). The research project by Parr *et al* (1997) explored the consequences and significance of acquired language impairment from the perspective of the people who have it. The study set out to examine the personal perspectives on aphasia within a social, economic and political context. Fifty people with long-term aphasia took part in in-depth interviews in which they described the onset of aphasia; its consequences for employment, education, leisure and social life and personal relationships; their access to information; their experience and evaluation of health, welfare and social care services; their perceptions and understanding of disability.

The findings from this qualitative study indicated that aphasia is experienced as a complex, dynamic process which influences every domain of social functioning, and affects the individual at a number of different levels – as someone who interacts with others, as a member of groups and communities, and as a citizen. This accords with the

11

description of aphasia as a multi-party system given by Goodwin (1995) and cited earlier in this chapter. In addition, the study detailed the disabling barriers that are faced by people with aphasia. For example, access to employment and educational opportunities is often restricted, and financial difficulties are not uncommon as a result. For many people with aphasia, authority and versatility of response in their relationships with others diminishes. Many people who have aphasia become isolated, and find it difficult to identify and join with others.

From the perspective of those who have it, aphasia makes itself felt, not just as an acute and traumatic event, but continuously as life events unfold. Family troubles and celebrations continue to expose the aphasia sometimes years after onset. Aphasia has a direct impact on the lives of the people who have it, but also compromises their negotiation of support and services. Access to relevant information is restricted for people who have difficulty understanding spoken and written language, and who may not be able to enquire or ask questions. In addition, people with aphasia create unique and idiosyncratic accounts of their impairment which change as the years pass, drawing on personal and cultural health-beliefs, the information that they have been able to access, and dominant models and influences. Each person proceeds through the experience of aphasia in a unique and unpredictable manner, rather than moving through a set of sequential and ordered stages. The intangible, invisible nature of aphasia means that it can be difficult to understand, even for those who live with it.

Issues of empowerment and emancipation

Issues of empowerment and emancipation form a central preoccupation of social model philosophy. Traditional rehabilitation often centres upon maximising the impaired individual's independence. Some disability theorists have questioned this, asking 'what is so important about independence?':

Health and welfare professionals usually regard independence as a central aim in the rehabilitation process. Disabled people define independence, not in physical terms, but in terms of control. People who are almost totally dependent upon others, in a physical sense,

> can still have independence of thought and action, enabling them to take full and active charge of their lives. Narrowly defined, independence can give rise to inefficiency and stress, as well as wasting precious time. (French, 1994, p47)

The disability movement places a higher value upon autonomy than upon independence. Disabled people may not aspire to do everything for themselves (an assumption which may underpin rehabilitation) but rather should be able to control the type and timing of the assistance they receive in order to achieve what they want.

Control of the nature and timing of assistance constitutes a form of empowerment that occurs at the level of personal autonomy. Social model theorists argue that rehabilitation professionals and services should act as a resource to this end (Jordan, 1998). However, such personal empowerment also takes place within the context of the political empowerment of disabled people as a whole. This is not without its complications, given the diversity of impairments and the different ways in which people experience them. There is evidence of increasingly radical activity by disabled people, however, and the charities and voluntary associations which represent them are being influenced by these developments. Thus, the UK-based charity Action for Dysphasic Adults (ADA) set up a working party of people with aphasia to look at the implications of the Disability Discrimination Act (which was passed in the UK in 1995) for those who have acquired language impairment. The resulting document, 'Open Hole the Stony Wall' has been sent to various Government ministers working within health, social care and welfare departments in the UK (ADA Working Party, 1998).

This initiative and others undertaken by groups of people with different impairments represent not just *empowerment* (in that disabled people are setting their own agenda and tackling the issues which concern them) but *emancipation*, in the sense that they are seeking to change existing policies, practices and structures. Again, it is important not to confuse these developments with the concept of independence. It is increasingly common for disabled people to use advocates in the pursuit of their aims. In the case of people with aphasia, advocates may have a crucial role in clarifying information, enabling choices and decisions, and representing their client's views and wishes. Self-advocacy is also increasingly in evidence. This is usually a collective process of gathering information, asserting rights and celebrating difference.

The relationship between impairment and disability

This issue is by no means straightforward, and has been the subject of a number of debates and discussions within the disability literature. Some disability theorists have pointed out that understanding disability purely in terms of social barriers effectively denies the existence and impact of the impairment. This argument is made with reference to states such as fatigue or pain, which are often experienced as an intrinsic part of an impairment, and which cannot be conceptualised in terms of socially constructed barriers (Crow, 1992).

In the process of attempting to accommodate the social model of disability, the World Health Organisation developed the so-called 'bridged' model of disablement (http://www.who.ch/icidh). This model, which remains in draft format, incorporates the idea of social barriers, but does not deny the existence of the impairment, nor the potential contribution of medicine (*see* Table 1.2).

It is not yet clear how disability theorists react to these suggestions. For some, proper consideration of impairment cannot come swiftly

Table 1.2 *The 'bridged' model of disablement*

Personal problem	AND	Social problem
Medical care	AND	Biopsychosocial integration
Individual treatment	AND	Social action
Professional help	AND	Individual and collective responsibility
Personal adjustment	AND	Environmental manipulation
Behaviour	AND	Attitude
Care	AND	Human rights
Health care policy	AND	Politics
Individual adaptation	AND	Social change

Source: WHO, 1999

enough. Hughes and Paterson (1997) argue that the existing social model of disability abandons or 'disembodies' impairment, leaving it entirely within the medical domain. They point out that while impairment is undoubtedly a physical phenomenon, it is also experienced as a cultural and social event. A sociology of impairment urgently needs to be developed. Drawing on post-modernist philosophies, they suggest that the experience of impairment needs to be deconstructed. Studies within narrative medicine are also highlighting the fact that, while the manifestation of disease or illness may take a standard physiological form, personal experiences are not homogenous. Interpretations of illness are essentially diverse and idiosyncratic, and shaped by cultural influences (Frank, 1995; Greenhalgh & Hurwitz, 1999).

This suggestion accords with the findings from the research by Parr *et al* (1997) which showed that people experience and interpret aphasia in diverse ways. Many people who have aphasia are preoccupied with their impairment, and are only concerned to see it improve and to make the best recovery possible. For some people, at certain times, issues of disability may seem irrelevant. This may be due to the fact that aphasia is a suddenly acquired impairment, often associated with acute illness. It may change, but often does not go away. Many people find it hard to acknowledge that, once the initial recovery has taken place, their aphasia is with them for life.

The study showed that people with aphasia experience numerous disabling barriers, as already described, but suggested that the removal of such barriers would not entirely lessen the impact of the impairment. The social barrier model, in this case, does not adequately describe the intrinsically disabling nature of language impairment that, for example, can compromise the individual's access to autonomy, negotiation, celebration and secrecy.

Putting theory into practice: a framework for aphasia therapy
The work of the aphasia centre is much influenced by the social model of disability, but also by developments within therapeutic and theoretical approaches to aphasia. We attempt to offer the person with aphasia a range of therapies, some of which directly address the impairment and

some of which address their disability from a social model perspective. The experience of aphasia is therefore seen as a multi-dimensional process. It is a priority to understand where each client is within this process, to try to ascertain how the client understands what has happened and what the outlook is, and to offer appropriate, relevant and useful choices and combinations within therapy.

Byng *et al* (in press) have developed a framework for therapy (*see* Figure 1.1) which depicts the multi-dimensional nature of aphasia and the different levels and types of therapeutic input which might be useful. In the next section of this chapter we will describe this model in detail, and use it to summarise the range of therapies offered at the aphasia centre.

The person with aphasia as a social being

In recent years, scientific investigation and clinical work with people who have aphasia have augmented a considerable body of knowledge concerning how aphasia affects language processing mechanisms (for

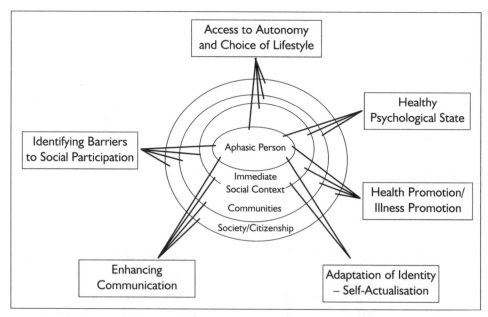

Figure 1.1 *Living with aphasia: goals of intervention* (**Source:** *Byng* et al, *in press)*

example, Thompson, 1998). Each individual with aphasia is now understood to display a specific constellation of impairments that affect the encoding and decoding of linguistic signals in particular ways. These can be investigated, tested, and described in detail. Meticulous analysis now underpins many impairment-based therapies – a related and worthwhile focus of clinical and research endeavour. Numerous single case studies have demonstrated that specific, rational therapies can overcome, or circumvent, aspects of language impairment (Helm-Estabrooks & Holland, 1998). It is hardly surprising that, from this perspective as from earlier clinical perspectives, people with aphasia are represented as 'cases', essentially defined in terms of their impairments.

Of course, therapists who undertake impairment-focused therapy are far from oblivious to the social consequences of language impairment, which are starting to be better understood. However, while some attention has been paid to the psychosocial corollaries of aphasia (Brumfitt, 1993; Le Dorze & Brassard, 1995) there has been comparatively little development in therapeutic approaches to psychosocial difficulties, beyond attention to the psychological well-being of the aphasic individual and that of the family (Ireland & Wotton, 1996; Hoen et al, 1997; Wahrborg et al, 1997).

Nevertheless, constructions of aphasia are shifting. Increasingly, aphasia is being described in terms of a collaborative process, rather than a neuropsychological state. For example, focusing on expressive language, Goodwin (1995) gives an elegant and discursive account of 'co-construction' in aphasia. He traces the elaborate process whereby the partner and nurse of a man with severe aphasia (Rob) painstakingly interpret his use of the three words which constitute his entire vocabulary ('yes', 'no' and 'and') together with his use of intonation, timing and body language, in order to find out what he wants for breakfast. This process is described as a 'tortured collaborative walk through contested taxonomic space'. Goodwin concludes:

If he could have said as simple a phrase as 'English muffin' all of the work examined here would have been unnecessary. However, the events investigated here do call into question traditional assessments

> of competence based purely on the ability to produce language. When Rob was in the hospital, his doctors, focused entirely on the trauma within his brain, said that any therapy would be merely cosmetic and a waste of time, since the underlying brain injury could not be remedied. Nothing could have been further from the truth, and medical advice based on such a view of the problem can cause irreparable harm to patients such as Rob and their families. (Goodwin, 1995, p31)

Clinicians and researchers such as Kagan (1998) and Simmons-Mackie (1998) have contributed to this sophisticated representation of aphasia, not as a discrete, circumscribed, autonomous neurolinguistic state, but as a systemic process which involves numerous players in constructing and negotiating meaning. In other words, their attention is drawn not only to the impairment itself, but beyond aphasia to the behaviour, responses and language of other people. The person with aphasia is not a solo performer, but part of a company of players. Specific therapies focus on enabling those in the aphasic person's orbit to reveal and acknowledge the competence of the linguistically impaired person (Kagan, 1998). To a certain extent, these developments break with traditional medical, linguistic and psychological constructions of aphasia and bring it within the domain of sociology and disability theory (Parr & Byng, in press).

However, it may be too restrictive to see aphasia simply in terms of intimate interactions. Aphasia does not just involve those within the aphasic person's immediate environment – caregivers, partners, friends and family members. In fact, the accounts and narratives given by people with aphasia suggest that they continue as participants (albeit compromised) within numerous intricate and intersecting social systems. Interacting with friends and family, people with aphasia are also members of institutions and communities, consumers of goods and services, and citizens in the broadest sense. This understanding of the person with aphasia as a complex social being is not at odds with social model theory, which switches attention from the impairment of the individual to disabling, socially constructed barriers.

It is desirable that any framework for therapy should have at its core a multi-faceted social being: the person with aphasia. In the model developed by Byng *et al* (in press) (*see* Figure 1.1), the person with aphasia is depicted as being the centre of a set of concentric and encompassing circles. These represent the individual surrounded by those in the immediate environment, a part of different communities and institutions (work, neighbourhood, church, school community) and finally as a citizen with rights and responsibilities.

Goals for therapeutic intervention

The framework developed by Byng *et al* (in press) depicts six main interconnected goals of therapeutic intervention in aphasia (each of which encompasses work currently ongoing or in development at the centre). These goals emerge from a number of sources, including therapeutic tradition, the principles of the social model of disability and current developments in healthcare policy. Each can be broken down into components of therapeutic intervention, some of which are well established in current clinical practice, others which are as yet innovative and tentative. The six interrelated goals of therapy are:

• Enhancing communication
• Identifying and dismantling barriers to social participation
• Adaptation of identity
• Promoting a healthy psychological state
• Promoting autonomy and choice
• Health promotion/illness prevention

Byng *et al* (in press) point out the essential interconnectedness of this model. Different goals may be addressed at the different levels of social functioning depicted. Thus, the goal of health promotion may be approached through working with the individual, with immediate interactants, with the different communities and institutions of which the individual is part and at a broader societal level through advocacy and education. Sometimes one major goal may provide a means of addressing another. Thus enhancing communication may itself be the major goal of intervention, or may be a means of addressing health promotion, or breaking down barriers. The components of each of the major goals are broken down in Table 1.3 and again demonstrate the interconnectedness of the model. Thus, components/

Table 1.3	Interventions designed to address the major goals of therapy in aphasia			
Goals of intervention	Examples of intervention programmes (not an exclusive or exhaustive list)			
	Individual	Immediate social context	Communities	Society/ Citizenship
Enhancing communication	• Therapies to improve language processing • Communication strategies • Conversation skills • Assertiveness training	• Enhancing communication skills of caregivers • Supported conversation	• Conversation partners	• Educational packages
Adaptation of identity	• Self-advocacy • Personal portfolios • Counselling • Self-help groups	• Enhancing communication • Counselling • Caregivers' groups	• Conversation groups • Creative arts groups	

Access to autonomy and choice of lifestyle	• Access to information • Personal portfolios • Enhancing communication • Self-advocacy	• Enhancing communication • Access to information	• Educational packages for employers, leisure and educational service providers, etc	• Information • Education packages for policy makers, social and healthcare service providers
Identifying barriers to social participation	• Provision of accessible information • Self-advocacy • Use of technology	• Enhancing communication	• Advocacy • Conversation groups	• Environmental modifications • Educational and training packages • Campaigning
Healthy psychological state	• Counselling • Pharmacological interventions • Self-advocacy • Psychotherapy	• Pharmacological interventions • Psychotherapy • Family therapy • Counselling	• Access to information • Support for differential diagnosis	
Health promotion/ illness prevention	• Stress management • Self-assertiveness • Enhancing communication	• Caregivers' groups	• Information and educational packages and training for service providers	• Information and educational packages for service providers

Source: Byng et al, in press

activities such as self-advocacy may be implemented in working towards several different goals, such as breaking down barriers, enhancing communication and promoting autonomy and choice.

Enhancing communication

This goal is perhaps the most familiar to therapists and has certainly in the past attracted the lion's share of therapeutic energy. Byng *et al* (in press) define the goal in terms of: 'achieving maximum potential by enhancing both the communication skills of the person with aphasia and the skills of those with whom they communicate'. Working towards this goal may involve a number of therapeutic activities including direct, impairment-focused therapies; development of compensatory communication strategies; training of conversation partners and enhancing the communication skills of those in the immediate environment.

Identifying and dismantling barriers to social participation

This goal is clearly much influenced by social model theory. Trying to practise what we preach, albeit not always successfully, we have become all too aware of disabling barriers within our own institutional procedures and practices. For example, if a person with aphasia is employed at the centre (and people have taken up various forms of employment including counselling, teaching, consultancy and research) the working environment and working procedures may need to be adapted. Thus, meetings can be made more accessible in terms of timing (perhaps short sessions with frequent breaks, or arranged for a time when participants are likely to be less tired, or taken slowly, with plenty of recapping and revision); decisions reached may need frequent verification and revisiting; minutes of meetings may need to be short, to the point and comprehensible. Changes such as these are not always easy to achieve or to sustain, especially when time is at a premium and a lot has to be accomplished. The student therapists who work at the centre gain first-hand experience of making structures explicit and accessible on a day-to-day basis. Streamlining the minutes of group meetings, for example, takes considerable amounts of time, thought and work even though the end impression is one of simplicity (*see* Figure 1.2 on pp24–5).

Adaptation of identity

This goal reflects the importance attached within the social model to issues of personal, social and collective identity. While interventions are, as yet, tentative and exploratory in nature, they involve supporting the person with aphasia in reconnecting with the 'pre-aphasic self', but in also establishing a strong, disabled identity, acknowledging and celebrating difference, connecting with communities and institutions, and developing a collective awareness of others with aphasia and the issues faced in common. Identity-focused therapy also accords strongly with the increasing interest in narrative-based medicine (Greenhalgh & Hurwitz, 1999), narrative being seen as the way in which individuals construct the embodied experience of illness and impairment and adjust their personal biographies accordingly. Working towards such a goal may involve a range of activities: for example, self-advocacy, groupwork, portfolio work, counselling and family therapy. The integrity of each of these activities is dependent upon the clinician's willingness and ability to listen to the story being told by the person with aphasia.

Promoting a healthy psychological state

Again, this issue is well covered in the existing literature and forms a part of current practice in aphasia therapy. A range of therapeutic interventions may be appropriate, including counselling (Ireland & Wotton, 1996), family therapy (Nichols *et al*, 1996), psychotherapy and pharmacological treatments for endogenous and reactive depressions (Andersen, 1997). At the aphasia centre, we are fortunate to have the services of Harry Clarke and Sue Boazman, who are employed as counsellors for clients and caregivers. Harry and Sue are members of a small group of counsellors in the United Kingdom who have personal experience of stroke and aphasia. They work closely with therapists at the centre in order to support the communication of clients, and to find the means of enabling them to disclose their worries and concerns (Clarke, 1998; Boazman, 1999).

Promoting autonomy and choice

This goal is clearly related to social model principles, in the sense that autonomy, control and choice are valued over 'functional independence'. It also accords with recent healthcare policy initiatives which seek to

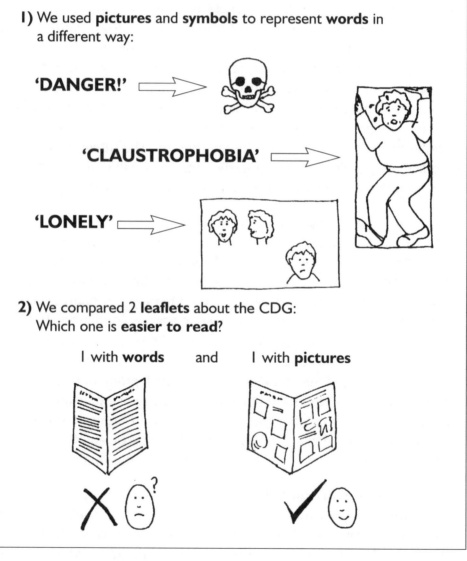

Minutes of 'Living with Aphasia' Group
Friday 20th November 1998

Group members: Peter, John, Sally, Rob, Jenny, Tom, Liz, Sam and Debbie

1) We used **pictures** and **symbols** to represent **words** in a different way:

'DANGER!' $\Longrightarrow$

'CLAUSTROPHOBIA' $\Longrightarrow$

'LONELY' $\Longrightarrow$

2) We compared 2 **leaflets** about the CDG: Which one is **easier to read**?

1 with **words**   and   1 with **pictures**

Figure 1.2 *An example of aphasia-friendly minutes*

3) Break.

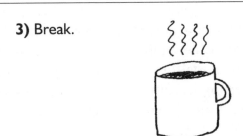

4) We **translated** part of a leaflet about Housing, to make it more **'aphasia-friendly'**.

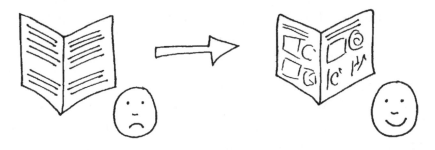

5) Next week: other ways of **getting information**.

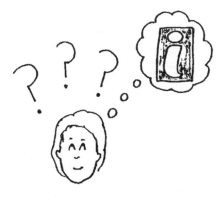

Figure 1.2 *continued*

promote informed choice and shared decision making (Coulter, 1997). The principle of promoting choices and decisions about therapy and about other issues is, as far as possible, embodied in the day-to-day running of the centre. Working towards this goal within therapy may involve a range of activities: for example, self-advocacy, identifying and dismantling barriers, assertiveness training, counselling, providing and campaigning for accessible information. This is clearly a critical issue for those whose written and spoken language is compromised.

Researchers and therapists at the centre, in conjunction with people with aphasia and other experts have recently developed *The Aphasia Handbook* (Parr *et al*, 1999). This is an information resource covering a wide range of medical and other topics, and written and presented in a style which makes it accessible to people with aphasia. It is hoped that this experimental resource will prove useful to those negotiating the maze of services and benefits.

Health promotion/Illness prevention

The work of therapists is increasingly understood in terms of promoting good health and preventing illness (Levenson & Farrell, 1998). Relevant interventions might concern preparing people for situations which they find difficult – for example, through assertiveness training and stress management. Health promotion and illness prevention are not just important for people with aphasia, but also for caregivers, whose knock-on health problems are well documented in the literature. We aim to support, inform and advocate for clients, where necessary. We promote an ethos of self-advocacy, and attempt to put clients in touch with relevant agencies and services. As far as possible, we try to support them in taking control of their own health.

An overview of therapy aims, while clarifying the range of interventions offered, invariably simplifies the process of working with each client to establish which package of therapy is most suitable at which time. Indeed, timing is a crucial aspect of the decision making regarding the choice and combination of therapies, interventions and support. For some people at a particular point in time, work on the impairment is the priority. Others may choose to address other aspects of living with aphasia. Figure 1.3 highlights

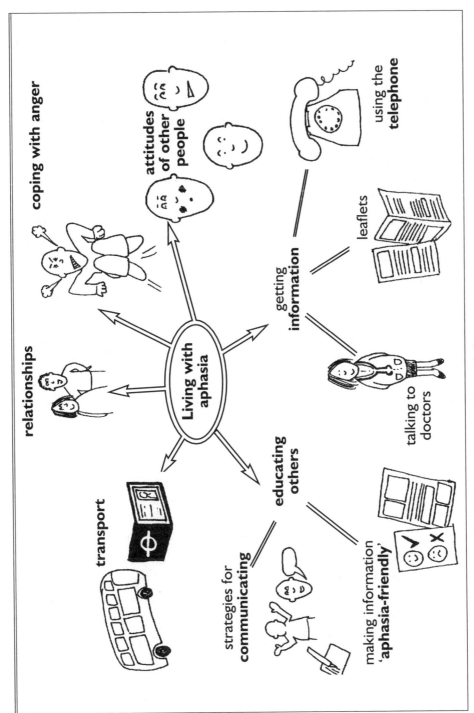

Figure 1.3 *Issues addressed in the 'Living with Aphasia' Group*

some of the issues covered in the Living with Aphasia Group. Some choose to tackle both the impairment and disability. The therapies and interventions can often work at the level of impairment and disability simultaneously. Thus, it may be perfectly possible for a client to work at improving skills in repairing conversation breakdowns, while a conversation partner is working towards improving the support for communication which can be offered.

Organising and delivering the service

At the aphasia centre we aim to offer an integrated range of therapy, support and training services which best meet the needs of the person with aphasia, their friends, relatives and others with whom they come into regular contact. Pathways through the range of therapeutic options inevitably differ according to the individual needs, preferences and circumstances of people who come to the centre.

Some people may come to the centre for several years of therapy while others will directly access only one of our social support groups or perhaps just the counselling service. For some people, the priority in therapy will be gaining support for the caregiver. Others find that their relatives are unable to be directly involved in sessions due to work and other family commitments, or difficulty travelling. Some people who leave the therapy groups do not return, while others come back regularly to attend one of the social groups or to help out with volunteer training and focus groups. The overriding principle is one of choice and flexible access to therapy, support, training and research. In Tables 1.4 and 1.5, we compare the weekly timetables of two different clients attending the centre.

The broad aims of the therapy groups are typically negotiated by clients and therapists on a termly basis. Being as explicit as possible about the aims of the groups is important; clients consider what they hear about the groups and indicate those they wish to join. They also identify the best slots of the day for individual sessions or, if requested, counselling input. Individual sessions with a keyworker will also provide the point of reference for monitoring of long- and short-term goals (described in Chapter 2) and evaluating the benefits and carryover from group sessions. Progress is regularly reviewed on a collaborative basis. Usually this involves discussion of future directions and negotiation of the leaving of therapy. This process is described more fully in Chapter 6.

Table 1.4 *Client 1: A typical week's therapy programme*

Time	Monday	Friday
10.30–11.30	**Group session** Storytelling Group • Word-finding strategies • Understanding the nature of the impairment	**Group session** Information Group • Developing aphasia-friendly poster • Access to services
11.30–11.45	**Coffee**	**Coffee**
11.45–12.30	**Individual session** • Writing skills • Developing a CV	**As above**
12.30–1.30	**Lunch**	**Lunch**
1.30–2.15	**Group session** Access to technology • Exploring e-mail and Internet • Telephone aids	**Group session** Coping with stress • Effects of stress on body/communication • Identifying stressful situations
2.15–3.00	Access to technology • Practical session	Coping with stress • Practising strategies

Ongoing support

People who leave the therapy groups or who access the centre looking for social outlets and increased opportunities for conversation may choose to come to one of our on-site support groups. These include: the *Conversation Group* (in which topical issues are discussed in conversations led by people with aphasia); the *Self-Advocacy Group* (which meets monthly and addresses more political issues); and the *Young People's Group* (which meets to discuss issues of particular relevance to young people who have had strokes and brain injury).

Table 1.5 *Client 2: A typical week's therapy programme*

Time	Monday	Friday
10.30–11.30	**Group session** Developing drawing skills • Categorisation tasks • Using enlargement techniques	**Group session** Video project – aphasia and competence • Demonstrating competence • Explaining aphasia
11.30–11.45	**Coffee**	**Coffee**
11.45–12.30	**Group session** Project work – using Total Communication in everyday environments • Pub outing	**Group session** Video project • Identifying what others can do • Filming
12.30–1.30	**Lunch**	**Lunch**
1.30–2.15	**Individual session** Counselling	**Group session** Working with relatives • Training conversation partners
2.15–3.00	**Group session** Conversation skills	**Group session** Working with relatives • Relaxation techniques

By the time people leave the centre, they have often accessed other forms of support and recreation in their area, such as a self-help group or local disability interest groups. Indeed, building such contact is an explicit part of the process of leaving therapy. If clients appear at risk of becoming isolated, ongoing support might involve the training of a volunteer who can visit the person in his or her home for supported conversation and visits to places of personal significance in the local community.

A further way in which we maintain a supportive contact with former clients is by inviting them to participate in regular volunteer and student training sessions and through participation in focus groups and feedback sessions relating to new developments and research projects.

Changing the ethos: environment, attitude and language

While offering direct therapies and interventions, we aim to create an ethos in which people who have aphasia and their families will feel comfortable, acknowledged and valued. This manifests itself in numerous ways – for example, in the welcoming and non-clinical atmosphere, the provision of informal seating areas, an accessible environment, freshly made snacks and sandwiches, and the friendly approach of staff and students.

As part of the endeavour to promote a non-clinical ethos, and mindful of the processes of co-construction, staff and students pay particular attention to the language and terminology they use. While running the risk of pedantic political correctness, we have become increasingly aware of the power of dominant discourses in disability (Corker & French, 1999). Given the predominantly medical culture of aphasia therapy, it becomes an ongoing challenge to scrutinise our own language and terminologies. Those who attend the centre are 'clients' or 'group members' rather than 'patients'. Rather than being 'discharged', they 'leave therapy'. Rather than being 'treated', they become partners in the therapy and goal-planning process, and develop their skills as group members. We also try to pay attention to problematising and passivising language, although this is not always easy either to identify or to replace, as many readers will be aware.

Conclusion

Working with people who have aphasia to provide therapies which they feel to be relevant and useful and to support their linguistic, psychological and social recovery in the longer term is a rewarding process, but is also fraught with difficulties and dilemmas. The process of ascertaining people's needs and priorities, developing with them a suitable package of therapies, listening to feedback and organising evaluation takes place within a context of constant concern about limited resources in terms of space and personnel.

While the interventions offered at the centre may appear similar to traditional therapies, we believe that they are different, both conceptually and in terms of how they are delivered. In discussing these issues – the foundation, implementation and implications of therapies for living with aphasia – we hope that this book will not only be useful in a practical sense but will offer therapists an opportunity for reflection and debate.

CHAPTER 2

Partnerships and Practicalities: Groupwork, Goal Setting and Evaluation

IN THIS BOOK we start to unpick some of the practice at the aphasia centre. This chapter begins with a discussion of some of the principles underlying the therapeutic interventions offered, with a particular focus on groupwork. We then describe the centre's approach to collaborative goal planning and evaluation – processes which are fundamental and will be revisited a number of times throughout this text.

Group therapy
Most of the people who attend the centre take part in groupwork. This continues a long-established tradition and constitutes a commitment to an effective form of intervention. While there are relatively few published investigations of the efficacy of group therapy for aphasia, changes in communicative ability in response to group intervention have been reported (for example, Aten *et al*, 1982; Bollinger *et al*, 1993; Sacchett *et al*, 1999; Elman & Bernstein-Ellis, 1999a). Groupwork has also been shown to improve the psychological well-being of aphasic people (Hoen *et al*, 1997; Brumfitt & Sheeran, 1997) and was an important feature of a project that addressed self-advocacy (Penman, 1998).

Elman (1999) reports a recent rekindling of interest in group intervention. While it is apparent that some of this interest stems from changes in funding for healthcare provision (faced with dwindling resources, some may consider groups to be more cost-efficient than individual therapy), it may also arise from the emergence of well documented and clinically relevant methods. The work of Kagan and her colleagues particularly springs to mind (Kagan & Gailey, 1993; Kagan, 1998; Kagan & Cohen-Schneider, 1999). In exploring the attractions of group therapy, these and other authors describe a number of communicative, psychosocial and performance-related benefits. These are elaborated in Table 2.1.

Different types of groups may enjoy different benefits. For example, therapy aimed at establishing communicative gesture may primarily exploit the opportunities for communication that accompany groupwork, while a self-advocacy forum may draw upon associated psychosocial benefits. Advancing the case for group intervention does not dismiss or downplay the contribution of therapy for aphasia on an individual basis. In fact, we see these approaches as complementary. Although groupwork is an important feature of our service delivery, our clients can also access a sizeable amount of individually based therapy. Each person attending the main therapy groups ordinarily participates in one additional session of individual therapy per week. A further clinical day per week is devoted to working with other clients for whom ongoing, one-to-one intervention seems more suitable.

Group or individual work? Selecting the therapeutic approach

The decision whether a client will work primarily in a group or in individual therapy is based on a range of factors, including their own skills, needs and preferences:

Clients who appear suited to *group therapy* at the centre:

- Have communication skills that include, at least, some reliable means of indicating 'yes' and 'no', and a way of conveying basic information (for example, wants and emotions) to therapy staff and other group members.

Table 2.1 *The benefits conferred by group therapy*

Benefit	Examples of benefit
Communicative	• A safe environment in which to experiment with new communication techniques (Fawcus, 1992) • Multiple opportunities to communicate with different partners (Davis & Wilcox, 1985; Fawcus, 1992) • Opportunities to witness, comment upon and learn from the communication attempts of others (Whitaker, 1989) • Provision of peer feedback regarding the intelligibility and effectiveness of communication (Elman & Bernstein-Ellis, 1999b) • Naturally arising and varied interactions (Kagan & Gailey, 1993; Elman & Bernstein-Ellis, 1999b) • An environment that (through exposure to a range of communication partners and situations) may promote generalisation of skill to non-clinical settings (Kearns, 1986; Elman & Bernstein-Ellis, 1999b)
Psychosocial	• Social re-engagement and companionship (Nichols & Jenkinson, 1991; Kagan & Gailey, 1993) • Sharing, discussion and joint problem solving of commonly experienced difficulties (Nichols & Jenkinson, 1991; Penman, 1998) • Peer support and empathy (Davis & Wilcox, 1985; Elman & Bernstein-Ellis, 1999b) • An environment in which to experiment with social roles and explore identity (Fawcus, 1989; Penman, 1998)
Performance	• Increased levels of arousal and participation, in response to the presence of an 'audience' (Fawcus, 1992) • Motivation by peers (Elman & Bernstein-Ellis, 1999b) • Naturalistic patterns of reinforcement (Kearns, 1986)

- Are willing to engage in therapy that addresses the linguistic, communicative and psychosocial sequelae of aphasia, and have concerns and needs broadly in keeping with those of other group members.
- Demonstrate certain cognitive skills (for example, some insight into communicative strengths and weaknesses; an ability to attend to a group task for a 45-minute period; an ability to remember general themes in therapy on a week-to-week basis) compatible with participation in an aphasia group.
- Are willing to participate in therapy with other aphasic people, and are able to monitor speaker change in a group setting.
- Are able to participate in group therapy from 10.30 am to 3.00 pm, twice weekly, on a regular basis.
- Are not receiving a similar speech and language therapy service elsewhere.

Clients who appear suited to *individually based therapy* at the centre:

- Are willing to engage in therapy that addresses the linguistic, communicative and psychosocial sequelae of aphasia, but have needs that are different from other group members and/or require a type of therapy not currently offered within the therapy groups.
- Are not willing or able to participate in group therapy with other people who have aphasia.
- Are not able to attend group therapy from 10.30 am to 3.00 pm, twice weekly, on a regular basis (perhaps because they are easily fatigued or have transport difficulties).
- Are not receiving a similar speech and language therapy service elsewhere.

Clearly, the way in which our service is delivered (for example, frequency of contact and hours of work) may affect the type of therapy a client accesses. Some clients are unable to attend for two group therapy days per week, and may participate in a period of individual therapy instead. The very nature of group and individual therapy may also assist in the decision-making process. For example, while group therapy confers a range of benefits that may not be apparent in one-to-one sessions, it primarily addresses the collective needs of a number of people with aphasia. This requires a certain amount of robustness in terms of cognitive, communicative and interactive skill on the part of the group members. In contrast, individual therapy can be more readily tailored to personal requirements and the therapist is able to offer undivided attention to the client.

Certain types of intervention also fit most comfortably within a group or individual framework. In our experience, those focusing on communication and conversation are enhanced by the interaction and peer feedback that occur in groups. Work that focuses directly upon the language impairment, in which careful shaping of targeted strategies is crucial to therapeutic success, probably proceeds best within individual sessions.

Preparing to implement group therapy

Group content and form
Some thought needs to be given to client abilities, the focus of groupwork and the likely configuration of any group. So far, this chapter has primarily referred to groups that have a specific therapeutic focus and are mediated by healthcare professionals. These types of groups predominate at the centre and include the therapy groups for people with comparable levels of language impairment, as well as mixed-ability groups that focus on areas such as stress management and interpersonal relationships. In these groups, therapy is delivered in discernible units (for example, addressing Total Communication [see Chapter 3], relaxation, negotiation skills) and the therapist assumes a central role in devising and carrying out sessions that build group members' skills and meet therapeutic goals. However, some other groups at the centre operate more autonomously. These include the self-advocacy, conversation and self-help groups. Group members more obviously organise and guide these groups, while therapy staff keep a relatively low profile. Indeed, as will be apparent in Chapter 3, therapist involvement in these groups can sometimes be counterproductive.

Irrespective of whether a group is therapist- or client-led, an early decision needs to be made about the lifespan of the group (that is, when it will begin and end). At the centre, we are fortunate in that most therapy groups have few time constraints. Ongoing phases of therapy are offered, and clients participate for as long as there is associated communicative and psychosocial benefit. Other, more specific groups may be more temporally bound: a six-session relaxation group for clients and caregivers is one recent example. In our experience, defined-duration groups are useful if the therapy on offer is somewhat novel and experimental, or if there is an expectation that, after an initial period of therapist-led facilitation, group members will assume responsibility for continued group functioning (as with the self-advocacy group).

Group composition

Another decision to be taken before implementing group therapy is whether a system of closed or open membership will operate (Adair-Ewing, 1999). *Closed membership*, in which the same people attend for the group's duration and no newcomers join them, carries the benefit that group members encounter and move through each stage of group work at roughly the same time. A stable membership may facilitate greater openness between group members and lead to the airing and mutual solution of common problems (Luterman, 1991; Schneider-Corey & Corey, 1997). We find that groups that run for a short or defined period often work best with a closed membership.

Open group membership, on the other hand, is characterised by a certain amount of client 'turnover' during the group's lifespan:

> The group continues at the same time and at the same place, but members commit for differing amounts of time, resulting in multiple beginning and ending dates. (Adair-Ewing, 1999, p12)

Inevitably, this movement within the group has an effect on dynamics, as friendships are forged and lost, and different constellations of skill and personality exert their influence. With new members, some revisiting of previous themes in intervention may be required, affecting the group's progression through therapy. As Adair-Ewing (1999) points out, however, a certain amount of change may be useful in group therapy. For example, recapping therapy techniques may help to consolidate existing group members' skills and reveal their expertise. We agree that the benefits of open group membership counter many associated drawbacks, as long as a core group of experienced members is maintained to continue the therapeutic process.

As group dynamics may also be affected by group size and homogeneity, these aspects also require careful consideration. *Group size* will be determined, in part, by the content and purpose of intervention (Kearns, 1986). For example, a group that meets to engage in stimulating and satisfying conversations may benefit from the interactive opportunities provided by a large membership. A group exploring the potential of computers in communication may be better served by a smaller membership: fewer members may mean more 'hands-on' experience. Groups with a specific therapeutic focus may be limited in size by the availability of therapy staff. At the centre, each of the therapy groups ordinarily comprises eight people with aphasia and is ordinarily facilitated by at least two student therapists. This client-to-therapist ratio allows for flexible application and monitoring of therapeutic techniques, with one student assuming primary responsibility for keeping the group 'on task' and the other providing assistance (for example, reiterating instructions or assisting with communicative repair), as required.

Group homogeneity (or the lack of it) can also have implications for staffing. We find that more communicatively heterogeneous groups generally require more input from therapists. Therapists assume a key role in clarifying communication attempts and ensuring equal access to 'the floor'. Even in relatively homogenous groups, there will be some variation in members' ability to understand and respond to therapy tasks. The challenge to therapists becomes one of providing sufficient time and communicative support to ensure participation by less able members, without slowing therapy to the degree that others feel bored or alienated. Some suggestions for working with mixed-ability groups appear later in this chapter.

Group leadership

A final consideration before starting group therapy concerns leadership: specifically, who will assume responsibility for coordinating and facilitating group meetings on an ongoing basis. As with group size, decisions concerning group leadership will be influenced by the content and purpose of intervention. A distinction has already been made between therapist- and client-led groups with the latter, in particular, focusing on the self-help and social aspects of groupwork. The involvement of therapists in this type of group must be carefully considered, and the attendant benefits and risks weighed up. We, and others, have found that therapist involvement in some of the organisational and procedural aspects at the inception of the group (for example, organising accommodation or helping to elucidate the purpose and possible content of group meetings) can be very useful (Le May, 1993). We have also discovered that, prior to aphasia, clients may have had little exposure to working in groups. A steep learning curve may be faced as they grapple with a novel situation as well as the idiosyncrasies of their own and others' aphasia.

Prolonged involvement by therapists in self-help and other client-led groups, however, may be detrimental to group functioning. Some common pitfalls include the therapist assuming responsibility for key group roles (for example, group initiator or minute-taker) and a tendency for the group to defer to the therapist in decision making. Therapists working in conversation groups should also be aware of the effect that their presence can have upon interaction. Some features of institutional discourse (for example, the therapist being afforded certain rights to introduce topics, apportion turns and pursue responses [Lesser & Milroy, 1993]) may become apparent. These ways of working, once begun, may be difficult to modify. One way of circumventing some of these problems is to agree the nature of therapist participation – for example, negotiating the type of facilitation to be offered and length of involvement before the group becomes established. The group may also seek within its own membership to fill pivotal roles, such as chair or spokesperson. Some other means of balancing clients' and therapists' contributions in group work are discussed in the study of the conversation group (*see* Chapter 3).

Facilitating group therapy

Leadership style

Group therapy can provide a powerful context for change (Fawcus, 1992; Adair-Ewing, 1999). A safe environment in which to meet with peers, experiment with new techniques and achieve common goals can be an important first step in transforming everyday communication, relationships and opportunities. Successful group therapy is well planned and structured; this chapter has already shown how the therapist may 'set the scene' for groupwork. As crucially, therapist performance within sessions may influence the effectiveness of group therapy. The style of leadership that they adopt can have a significant impact upon group interaction.

Several authors have reported the benefits of achieving a *facilitatory* style in group therapy (Fawcus, 1992; Kagan & Gailey, 1993; Holland & Beeson, 1999). This method of leadership is associated with:

- A focus on the contributions of group members within therapy.
- Encouraging group members to share experiences and initiate exchanges.
- Associated efforts to minimise therapist contributions, other than those that clarify and summarise group proceedings.
- The provision of aphasia-friendly materials and communication techniques to enhance access to the conversational floor.
- Creating an environment in which the expression of different viewpoints is encouraged and respected.
- The use of peer monitoring and feedback as a vehicle to effect change.

Having observed a variety of leadership styles in our role as student trainers, and worked with groups ourselves, we would agree that a facilitative model fits group therapy well. In effective groups, members interact freely and truthfully, providing feedback about peers' communication and behaviour (Adair-Ewing, 1999). The facilitatory style, with its emphasis upon members' contributions and interaction, can encourage this type of group function. A more *didactic* style of leadership, in which therapist–client rather than client–client interactions predominate, seems less suited to groupwork. Indeed, Kearns (1986) comments:

> If a group leader sequentially treats each individual in a group, and there is little interaction other than individual exchanges between the

clinician and a given patient, the result may be inefficient individual treatment within a group setting. (Kearns, 1986, p313)

Promoting group interaction: setting the rules

While the use of a facilitatory style of leadership may promote group interaction, other steps are sometimes necessary to ensure consistent and equitable contributions by group members. Again, it is worth considering that members may have had limited exposure to groups. Working with others and, in particular, speaking out in a group context may be a new and anxiety-provoking experience for some. For this reason, it is often useful to set group rules at the start of therapy. These rules are often most relevant if generated by group members themselves. Asking members to reflect upon the features of 'good' as opposed to 'bad' groups may be an appropriate starting point. At the aphasia centre, group rules often address issues surrounding punctuality and attendance, encourage the use of Total Communication (*see* Chapter 3), and urge all members' contributions to group proceedings. An example of an agreed set of group ground rules is given in Figure 2.1.

Setting group rules is especially useful when working with groups of people with different levels of impairment and ability. Such groups may be more difficult to facilitate, largely because of some mismatch in members' communicative skills. A clear requirement for equal contributions, and the use of multimodal communication, may assist in creating more balanced access to the conversational floor. There will be times, however, when additional effort is needed to meet the needs of more and less communicatively able participants. It may be useful, for example, to break into two smaller groups for some activities, with each group completing a different task around the same theme. For example, if the therapy theme is communicative drawing (*see* Chapter 3), more able members may be asked to generate and draw three occupations, while less able participants may focus on drawing their most recent job. Group cohesion may be maintained by all members sharing their contributions at the end of the activity.

Some mismatch in ability can also have implications for the timing of therapy tasks. Too fast a pace risks alienating less able group members,

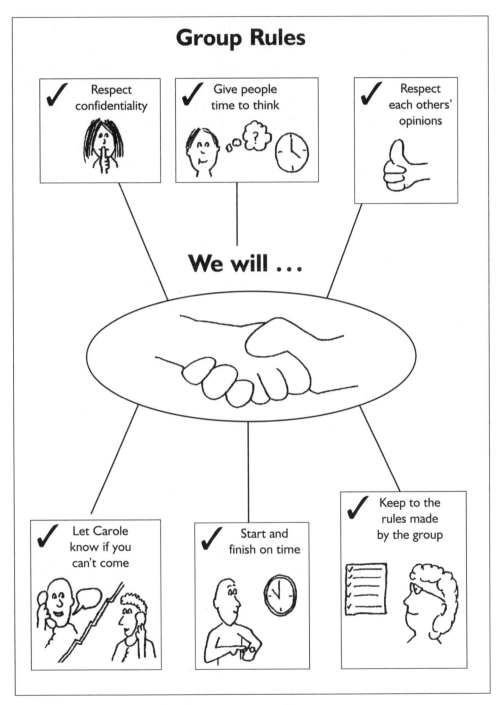

Figure 2.1 *An example of agreed ground rules*

while too slow a pace may irritate the more skilled. One way of dealing with this situation is for more able participants to take on additional responsibilities. As in the example above, these members may take on more in the allotted time. They may also be asked to assume certain roles (for example, as minute-taker) as well as complete group therapy tasks. Members who experience consistent difficulty in understanding and/or completing group activities may benefit from extra explanation of and practice in these aspects within individual therapy sessions.

The idea of assigning specific roles to designated group members can also be used to overcome problems related to non-participation. One severely aphasic client who comes to the centre became noticeably more engaged when asked to act as time-keeper during sessions. Another member's contributions increased when taking on the task of indicating 'who goes next' in group tasks. It is useful to note that the opportunity to experiment with different roles is viewed as one of the attractions of group therapy, and may be important in re-establishing identity (Fawcus, 1992; Penman, 1998).

Methods in group therapy

Throughout this book, detailed accounts will be given of therapy methods that can be used with groups. As a general guide, however, several techniques used in group therapy are outlined in Table 2.2.

Goal planning and evaluation: whose goals are they anyway?

Collaborative goal setting is an important part of our approach at the aphasia centre, and fits well within therapy informed by the social model of disability. This method of goal setting acknowledges the expertise that client and therapist bring to decisions about therapy, effectively combining insider accounts and experiences of aphasia with professional knowledge and perspectives. Indeed, the principle of shared decision making is incorporated within professional codes:

All episodes of care will be negotiated and agreed between client and carer and the speech and language therapist. (Royal College of Speech and Language Therapists, 1996, p22)

Table 2.2 *Some methods in group therapy*

Method	Description	Examples
Cohesion activities	Activities to gel new groups, or used as 'warm-up' tasks at the beginning of group meetings. A 'warm-up' task may also introduce the overall theme of therapy.	• Each member shares one piece of good news and one piece of bad news with the group. • (Before a session broaching *identity*) Clients are asked *'If you were an animal, what sort would you be and why?'*
Modelling	A therapist-led means of demonstrating behaviours, usually for comment or analysis by the group. Modelling may also be used to highlight and reinforce effective strategies.	• The therapist models a controlled breathing technique for use in stressful situations. • The therapist uses Total Communication in all interactions within the clinic.
Role play	Clients re-enact difficult, real-life scenarios for analysis and problem solving by the group. Role-play may also be used to test suggested solutions and new responses.	• A client acts out a recent, unsuccessful attempt at ordering food at the pub. After possible solutions are generated by the group, he uses communicative drawing in a further enactment.
Feedback	Therapist- or client-led comment upon others' performance. In order for feedback to be relevant and discriminate, clients need a clear description of which aspects of performance are to be observed.	• Clients watch a video of the group conversing. As they watch, they complete a checklist about turn taking. • Therapist and client use gesture in a PACE-style task. The watching group is asked if gesture helped in getting the message across.
Brainstorming	Clients are encouraged to generate as many solutions as possible to a given scenario. The relative merits of each solution are debated before one or two are chosen for modelling or role play.	• Clients brainstorm potential means of dealing with a difficult shop assistant when asking for a refund. One group member selects the 'broken record' approach to try in role play.

Source: Adapted from Hitchings (1992)

45

In addition to the principle of shared decision making, the manner in which decisions are made requires careful consideration. There are many potential barriers to achieving a genuinely shared control over the therapy process. These include the physical limitations caused by illness or disease; poor communication between healthcare practitioners and their clients; and limited opportunity to be involved in issues concerning care. As Maclaren (1996, p492) explains: 'rehabilitation practitioners need to be aware of the need for unbiased information giving, and the power they hold to subtly manipulate patient choices.' These points are highly relevant given that aphasia may make it more difficult to seek out and negotiate therapy, and to question and challenge providers. Services themselves may be experienced as disabling barriers, affecting individuals' control over key aspects of their lives (Finkelstein, 1991; Parr *et al*, 1997).

Horton *et al* (1998) carried out a survey that revealed some dissatisfaction among people with aphasia and caregivers regarding their degree of involvement in decisions about speech and language therapy. From evidence such as this, it seems that therapists' underlying concern to empower clients to share the therapy process may not always reflect service users' perspectives. Speech and language therapists may continue to find themselves in contexts in which the medical model is the dominant paradigm and in which limited resources may further impact upon the delivery and scope of therapy.

Traditionally, therapists commence their involvement with a thorough assessment of the client's speech and language, and communication abilities and needs. While this approach yields considerable information upon which to base intervention, it may also serve to reinforce the idea of the therapist as expert and the aphasic person as recipient of this expertise. Although speech and language therapists will routinely include some evaluation of the communicative environment, the emphasis may still be upon the pathology of the individual. Correspondingly, the focus of intervention may fall upon reducing the language impairment or improving the use of communication strategies. Of course, this type of therapy may be entirely appropriate, and negotiated between therapist and client. However, therapy may sometimes proceed with limited exploration of the client's everyday needs, wants and circumstances. This runs the risk of missing other important therapeutic endeavours (such as training conversation partners) and restricting client choice to more peripheral matters (such as the timing of appointments, or which of the impaired modalities to address in therapy). This may mean that the client experiences less than optimal control over the therapeutic process.

Within the traditions of more conventional assessment, it may also be that limited consideration is given to the barriers that prevent the individual from achieving personal autonomy. Often, they are omitted from goal planning; the section that follows will explain how exploration of these issues may take place. Again, therapy and the therapeutic process itself may constitute or reflect socially constructed barriers. Many people with aphasia are unsure about what to expect from speech and language therapy and come to therapy anticipating that the therapist will know what is best for them. This is particularly so in the early stages when the person is experiencing ill health and is, in a very real sense, a patient. As patients and practitioners ourselves, we have all witnessed at first hand how easy it is to assume a passive, dependent patient role in discussing and deciding upon medical and therapeutic interventions.

The nature of client–clinician relationships that stem from these earlier experiences can persist throughout the duration of contact with services, perhaps supported by the uneasy balance of power that tips in favour of the healthcare professional. An example of this is when clients who attempt to take greater control over their own care (perhaps by adapting or rejecting professional advice) become known as 'difficult', 'non-compliant' or 'unmotivated'. It has been, and sometimes remains, challenging for us as therapists to share control and responsibility for change with our clients. A shift in therapeutic relationships can only happen if therapists are willing to open subtly different dialogues with clients, which calls for:

---

changed understandings, new ideologies, new skills, new organisational structures, new relationships between those who serve and those who are served. (Tyne, 1994, p253)

A framework for collaborative goal setting: problem-focused goal planning

Problem-focused goal planning seems to be an approach that can assist in redressing the balance of power between therapist and client, as well as in identifying therapeutic aims which have genuine relevance and meaning to the person with aphasia. In this approach, therapist and client work in partnership through the process of identifying problem areas, setting goals and action plans, and evaluating the effectiveness of therapy, each person bringing an equally important but different kind of expertise to the relationship. The process of goal planning is seen not as an aid or precursor to the therapy, but as an integral part of the therapeutic process itself. Clients regain 'mastery over their own situation through informed decision making' (Maclaren, 1996 p497).

Problem-focused assessment

A major aspect of the problem-focused assessment is an in-depth interview. Before this is carried out, the therapist will spend time getting to know the client informally and assessing his or her communication. This is done in order to establish how best to optimise the client's communication during the interview. As with more traditional approaches, the starting point is almost always *an informal conversation* during which the therapist can observe the client's use of language and communication strategies, together with the response to different styles and levels of input, and to a range of facilitation techniques. These observations are extended as necessary by further informal or formal assessment of language and communication. Only when the therapist has sufficient understanding of the client's communication impairments and abilities to permit effective facilitation of that client's expression and comprehension can the interview be carried out.

Through the *interview process*, the therapist and client build up a shared understanding of the nature of the issues to be addressed in therapy. An open and honest dialogue allows them to gain insight into each other's perspectives. This can be a time-consuming process, particularly when the client's communication impairment is severe. It requires a degree of flexibility and reflection from both client and therapist. As such, it is generally more useful for therapists and clients working together in rehabilitation or community settings than for those in acute settings. In the early days of aphasia it may still be very difficult to identify the impact of the language impairment (although aspects of the problem-focused interview can be incorporated into assessment from the very early stages). The interview may take several sessions to carry out, and the therapist should use whatever communication strategies are necessary to facilitate the client's active participation. With the client's consent, a third person, such as a caregiver, relative or advocate, may often make a useful contribution to the interview process.

The initial interview carried out at the centre follows a semi-structured format. There are no set questions and the ordering of questions is not rigid, thus allowing the therapist to be flexible and responsive to the client, to provide and learn about appropriate support for communication, and allowing the client to raise any important issues or concerns. However, the therapist does use a topic guide to ensure that the client is given the opportunity to discuss a range of issues which may be important to people living with communication impairment (Parr *et al*, 1997; Communications Forum, 1998). Many of the topic areas covered will be familiar to speech and language therapists, but the initial interview is qualitatively different to taking a traditional case history. This is because the focus, rather than primarily falling on what the aphasic individual can and cannot do, is on the impact of aphasia on the individual's lifestyle. Communication is supported by a resource of pictographic and keyword information, some of which is drawn from the *Pictographic Communication Resources Manual* (Kagan *et al*, 1996) and some of which has been developed at the centre specifically for this purpose.

In the interview a number of key issues are explored in depth: the disabling barriers encountered, autonomy and control in decision making, and satisfaction with different aspects of life. During discussion, the therapist tries to find out from the clients about the environment in which they operate, the nature of the challenges faced and how these are dealt with, how far they feel they have control over their situation and what they would most like to change about life with aphasia. An example of a topic guide is given in Table 2.3. This is not intended to be prescriptive and may be adapted for use in other therapy settings.

Table 2.3 *Initial interview topic guide*

Major themes to be discussed in all the topic areas are: *barriers (external and internal); autonomy and dependence; control over situation; satisfaction with situation.*

Family and domestic situation
• Details; type of contact with other family members
• Caregiving responsibilities (who cares for client, for whom does client care)
• Present and past roles within family (breadwinner, homemaker, responsibility for household finances, etc)
• Social and welfare services' involvement

Social life
• Weekly pattern and networks
• Hobbies and interests
• Established and new relationships
• Choice over social contact

Occupation
• Type of occupation (past and present); paid/domestic/voluntary roles
• Aspirations

Financial issues
• Sources of income
• Benefits applied for/received
• Money worries

Health
• Long-standing health issues
• Current health concerns
• Health services (currently used or needed)

Communication
• History of communication difficulties
• Understanding of own impairment
• Own perceptions of current strengths and difficulties
• Uses of reading and writing (pre-aphasia and current)
• Functional independence
• Opportunities in daily life

Emotional well-being
• Responses to aphasia: client and others
• Perception of well-being: depression? stress and anxiety? frustration and anger?
• Coping styles
• Any other issues raised by client

The use of problem-focused assessment does not preclude the use of more *formal assessments* of speech, language and communication. These latter assessments and observations may help focus and plan impairment-based therapy or support the successful planning and implementation of other forms of therapy. For instance, it may be necessary to assess a client's comprehension of written words and sentences formally in order to know how best to present written information during therapy sessions or interviews. A clear understanding of a client's language impairments is necessary for the therapist to know which modalities and strategies might be available to that individual in therapy for developing Total Communication. A clear analysis of breakdown in language processing may support the development of accessible explanations about aphasia which may be central to therapies addressing identity (*see* Chapter 5).

Formal assessment may also be used to provide objective evidence of the effectiveness of particular therapies, where these specifically address aspects of language and communication. However, the assessment of the impairment should be carried out only as is directly relevant to the needs which have been identified as the focus of therapy, rather than carrying out a battery of assessments simply because it is the standard professional practice. As Finkelstein (1991) argues:

> The medical model and its rehabilitation service approach should always be determined in the context of the social (barriers) model and not vice versa … In effect, this means that the extent, duration and nature of medical interventions should be guided by an understanding and analysis of the barriers to be overcome, rather than on the functional limitations of the individual. (Finkelstein, 1991, pp35-36)

Identifying key problems

Chapter 1 described how the impact of aphasia on an individual's life is usually complex and far reaching, and the barriers encountered may be numerous. The issues raised at the initial interview will usually involve some problems that are amenable to change through speech and language therapy, some that can be addressed through other resources and services, and some that cannot effectively be addressed at an individual level (such as those dependent on political change or legislation). The issues that might be addressed within the broad scope of speech and language therapy may be too much to deal with within a time-limited intervention. It seems sensible, therefore, to identify key issues which become the main focus of therapy.

The identification of key problems again requires collaboration. It is often useful to create a shared record of the most important points raised during the interview, perhaps in keyword or pictorial form as required by the person with aphasia. Where possible, this should incorporate the language or images used by the client, since a direct record of what was expressed is often a more reliable means of identifying problems than translation through the wording of a therapist (Hay *et al*, 1979).

This both assists clear communication during the interview – for instance, by signalling immediately if there has been any misinterpretation – and provides a useful point of reference for subsequent work. For example, one client expressed her worries about her drop in finances since she had been unable to return to work following her stroke. This point might be recorded as shown in Figure 2.2.

When the interview is complete, the whole record can then be used to facilitate the client to indicate (through pointing or any means accessible to them) which of the identified issues are of key importance, while the therapist has the opportunity to give information about issues such as the range of services available locally, and the relative usefulness of different forms of intervention. Through a process of dialogue, client and therapist come to agree on a small number of key problems which both reflect the priorities of the client and can realistically be addressed through therapy. Although this process may at first sight appear slow and inefficient compared to a model in which the therapist more actively controls the assessment and the treatment approach, it can lead to time saving in other ways.

For instance, by identifying the key issues to be addressed in therapy from the start, the therapist can avoid carrying out too many detailed formal assessments which may later prove irrelevant to the therapy

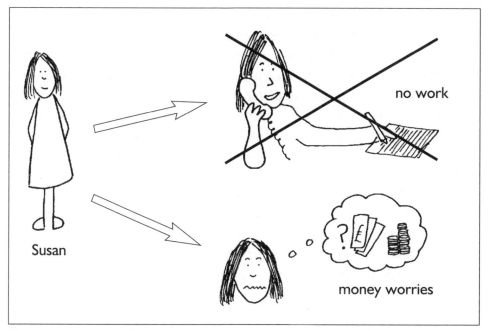

Figure 2.2 *Using client images to support goal planning*

actually undertaken. In addition, by informing the client openly and realistically from the outset about what therapy can and cannot achieve for them, the therapist is less likely to need to spend time addressing that client's unrealistic expectations at a later stage.

Problem-focused goals and action plans

There is a common misconception that the therapist who offers therapies for living with aphasia cannot seek to change the client's language processing or communication skills, but should only work to improve the disabling environment. As discussed elsewhere in this book, however, work on language and communication forms a key and vital part of the therapy approach that we are using at the centre. The way in which this approach differs from some more traditional aphasia therapy approaches is that the underlying principle is not necessarily the reduction of impairment per se, but rather *the reduction of the impact of the impairment on the client's lifestyle*. This is a subtle distinction and the difference may not always be immediately apparent. Thus, as the key problems identified in the problem-focused assessment are defined in terms of the impact of aphasia on the client's life and the barriers they encounter, the therapy goals will reflect steps towards reducing the impact of aphasia and/or assisting the client to overcome the barriers identified. However, in order to achieve these aims, goals may be set at any of the levels of impairment, disability or handicap/well-being. Depending on the individual's circumstances and perspectives a very different approach might be needed to address the impact of the 'same' aphasic problem. This can be illustrated by the following example.

A client (*John*) may identify a key problem in terms of his embarrassment when he cannot access familiar words, like family names. There are a number of ways in which John and the therapist might decide to address this problem. These might include:

- Cognitive neuropsychologically based therapy to improve access to a treated set of personal names and other relevant words.
- Development of a communication book, including photos of family members which John can point at to refer to someone who is not present in the room.
- Counselling to assist John in working through the emotional impact of the naming difficulty.
- Work with the family enabling them to support alternative forms of communication.

Thus it is perfectly justifiable to set therapy goals at an impairment level but only where therapist and client agree that this will be the most effective way of reducing the impact of the individual's aphasia and/or overcoming the barriers they face. Once the set of key problems has been agreed, the therapist and client can together draw up a goal and action plan. The goals set should relate directly and explicitly to the key problems, thus ensuring that the therapy will be relevant and meaningful to the client.

As with other approaches to goal setting, goals should be explicit, realistic, finite, measurable and time-bound. This ensures that therapist and client have a shared understanding of the intended outcomes of therapy, and permits a meaningful evaluation of its effects. The wording of goals should be explicit, client-centred and as far as possible be expressed in language that is accessible to the individual. For instance, in the example of John the goal might be: 'For John to be able to refer to his wife and children.' Once goals have been agreed, it becomes possible to formalise a therapy action plan. This is a written summary of what actions need to be taken in order to achieve each of the goals, who is responsible for carrying out the actions, and the time by which they should be completed. Using an action plan enables the therapist and client to know what they are each going to contribute during the therapy, and why they are carrying out particular activities, since these are explicitly related to the problems and goals identified. Of course, goal and action plans are not written in stone and can be adapted at any stage during the course of therapy. Indeed, it is often necessary to modify the plan if circumstances change, if the client's priorities shift, or if the identified goals prove unexpectedly difficult to achieve.

An example of a problem-focused approach to goal planning is given in Case Study 2.1.

Case Study 2.1 Melanie's life and Melanie's goals

Melanie, 33, lived with her teenage son and very supportive partner. She had worked part-time in her local hairdressers until a stroke 18 months previously had resulted in aphasia and weakness of her right arm and leg. The therapist who put her in touch with the centre reported the following features of her aphasia:

- Speech restricted to social phrases and a limited range of single words, mainly nouns.
- Ability to generate a wide range of written nouns, as well as some verbs and simple phrases. Although spelling was impaired, Melanie's written messages were usually clear in context.
- Ability to convey information effectively using drawing, gesture and a personalised communication book. However, Melanie was

reluctant to use these strategies with anyone outside her immediate family.

- Mild impairments of reading and auditory comprehension.

Following an initial visit to the centre, during which she spent a session in informal discussion with one of the centre therapists and also observed group activities, Melanie decided that she would like to join the group. Her initial interview took place over several sessions, and revealed a number of key issues. These included:

- General loss of confidence and self-esteem since the stroke.
- High level of anxiety about communicating with anyone outside the immediate family, with the result that Melanie tended to avoid any situations where she might be expected to communicate with unfamiliar people.
- Boredom and isolation due to unemployment, and also due to Melanie now having virtually no contact with her pre-stroke friends.
- Frustration associated with communication breakdown, with Melanie reporting that she was often unable to express herself clearly, and would tend to give up when her message was not understood.
- Dissatisfaction with her level of reliance on her partner and son to communicate for her and to fulfil aspects of her former role in the family, such as shopping and speaking to her son's teachers.

Melanie began attending a therapy group two days a week in which she participated in sessions on Total Communication (see Chapter 3), assertiveness, accessing information about benefits and project work. Together with her student keyworker, Melanie developed a problem-focused goal plan to guide work in weekly individual sessions. Her priority at this time was to be able to go shopping independently at her local shops. Melanie's goal plan is presented in Table 2.4.

Table 2.4 *Melanie's goal plan*

Long-term aims	For Melanie to feel more confident communicating with strangers For Melanie to be more independent of her family
Key problems	Melanie cannot always explain what she needs at a shop Melanie finds it difficult to understand numbers when a shopkeeper tells her the price Melanie feels anxious about how people will react to her communication difficulties when she goes shopping
Goals	1 For Melanie to be able to use strategies: • to explain her communication difficulties to strangers • to explain how people can help her to communicate • to ask for what she needs in a shop • to ask the shopkeeper to write down the price 2 For Melanie to feel confident enough to go shopping alone at her local newsagents
Actions	During individual sessions once a week for the Spring term: 1 Melanie and her keyworker will: • identify Total Communication strategies for each of the situations listed in Goal 1 • practise using these communication strategies in role play 2 Melanie and her keyworker will visit local shops where: • her keyworker will use the communication strategies with the shopkeeper • Melanie will observe how well the strategies work, and how the shopkeeper reacts 3 Melanie and her keyworker will visit several shops together where Melanie will try out the communication strategies 4 Melanie will try out the communication strategies on her own at the local newsagents

Group goal planning

Working within a group setting, the principles of goal setting are largely the same as those described for individual clients. Again, it is necessary to identify the key issues, agree explicit goals and summarise the steps to be taken towards achieving the goals. With regard to identifying problem areas, the in-depth interview is clearly less suitable for use with a group of people than with individuals. However, we have found that similar issues regarding the impact of aphasia and the barriers encountered tend to emerge naturally during group discussions, provided group members have the opportunity to initiate and develop topics according to their own interests. It is useful from time to time (such as at the end of a term or when the group membership changes) to set one or more therapy sessions aside for the group members to review the 'package' of therapy that they are involved in. At these times, the group members can discuss how each of the programmes is going, whether the goals have been met, and whether the therapy is still fulfilling a useful function. Changes in priorities can be identified through this process, and accommodated in the therapy.

The therapist's role at this stage can be described as follows:

- To create opportunities for the group to share experiences and concerns.
- To facilitate each group member's communication, supporting participation in the discussion.
- To assist the group in identifying common themes.
- To agree a plan which is relevant and meaningful to all group members.

We often find that it is useful to identify the general group aims in relation to a problem area shared by the group, and then to set individual goals related to these aims. For instance, a group may identify a common problem area of anxiety about summoning help if an emergency were to arise while group members were alone at home. This could translate into a general group aim for all members to have some means of summoning help in an emergency. Within this broad group aim, individual goals might vary from member to member:

- To be able to dial 999 and name the emergency service required.
- To have emergency messages recorded on a communication aid.
- To access information about a local personal alarm service in a format which is easy to understand.

In this way both the group members and the therapist share a clear understanding of the specific changes which should come about as a result of the group therapy.

Issues in evaluation – the role of the goal

In Chapter 6 we discuss the wider issues relating to evaluation and outcome measurement in therapies for living with aphasia, and explore methods of involving clients maximally in this process. In the following section we describe how goal planning can represent a flexible and important component of user-centred evaluation tools.

This approach to evaluation is based around the explicit problem-focused goal plan drawn up with each client and group. As already outlined, it is critical to ensure that the parameters that are measured are directly related to the clients' perceptions of their specific concerns and requirements. At the same time, the standard structure that is used for recording problems and goals permits us to make comparisons between very distinct therapies offered to individuals, and to gather information about the effectiveness of therapy across all our clients.

As with earlier stages in the goal-planning process, evaluation is carried out collaboratively between client and therapist. The areas that are considered in monitoring change are the problems and goals stated on the goal plan. We feel that it is important to ascertain our clients' subjective perceptions of change since these are the most meaningful indicators of how far they have benefited from therapy. As far as possible, we also back these subjective measures up with more objective ones.

Evaluating changes in clients' perceptions of problems

Since the primary focus of the goal plan is the identification of individual concerns that the therapy is intended to reduce, it makes sense that the evaluation of their perception of problems forms a vital part of evaluation of the therapy. This is done by asking the client to rate their perception of the severity of each problem before therapy and at the time of review. This approach is an adaptation of work by Mulhall (1978) and Shapiro (1961). Once the list of key problems has been agreed between client and therapist, the client is asked to rate how much each of the problems concerns them, using a seven-point visual analogue or 'faces' scale (adapted from Kunin, 1955). This rating is recorded on the goal plan and compared with ratings of the same problem statements at later times. Reduction by at least two points on the scale is taken to indicate that the problem is perceived to have diminished.

Wherever possible, these ratings are backed up by other forms of evidence that indicate the presence or severity of specific concerns. These other forms of evidence vary according to the nature of the problem being rated. For example, if a key problem relates to a client's lack of social opportunities associated with unemployment, then evidence that the client has commenced regular voluntary work or has re-established social contact with former work colleagues would be noted with their ratings of that problem after therapy. If the problem is one of anxiety about communicating with strangers then a communication stress questionnaire administered pre- and post-therapy may be used to provide more detailed evidence of change, in addition to the problem rating on the goal plan. If the problem is one that relates directly to the client's communication impairment, then evaluation may incorporate objective assessment of language and communication.

Of course, a numerical score on a simple rating scale is a simplistic measure of what may be a complex and multi-faceted problem. For this reason, any review of the problem ratings is followed by a more in-depth discussion to ascertain a fuller picture of the nature and attribution of any changes that have come about. Verbatim recording of a client's comments about an issue provides qualitative evidence which can carry as much weight as any rating scores.

Evaluating achievement of goals

The second major strand of evaluation occurs when therapist and client assess whether each of the goals on the goal plan has been achieved. In order for this to be possible, it is desirable for the wording of the goals to be explicit and either finite or measurable, as it may be impossible to know whether a loosely worded goal has actually been achieved. In order to provide some evidence of the outcomes of therapy, the success criteria related to each goal must also be made explicit at the outset. Some examples of success criteria might include demonstrable change in:

- Objective measures of language or communication ability
- Client's access to required services or information
- Client or caregiver knowledge
- Use of strategies in specific situations
- Opportunities for social interaction
- Confidence and self-esteem rating scales
- Development of a personalised communication book
- Satisfaction with a specific aspect of life as confirmed by the client and/or caregiver in a semi-structured interview.

Through this approach to therapy evaluation we suspect that it may be possible to tailor outcomes measurement so that it accurately reflects the specific nature of an individual client's therapy, but at the same time is carried out within a framework that allows for therapy to be evaluated similarly across a group of clients with widely differing concerns and requirements.

Groupwork, goal setting and evaluation are collaborative processes that are clearly dependent upon communication, yet many clients arrive at the centre with severely compromised language and communication skills. One of the first priorities is to develop with each client the best and most effective means of communication, and to support everyone concerned in using these. This endeavour forms the subject of Chapter 3.

CHAPTER 3

Facilitating Communication

Approaches to communication

Of the topics outlined in this book, therapists will perhaps be most familiar with communication. Traditional therapies for communication have focused on improving the aphasic person's use of verbal strategies such as circumlocution and/or non-verbal methods including gesture and drawing (Green, 1982; Trupe, 1986; Coelho, 1991; Rao, 1994). The client's ability to take turns and repair instances of communication breakdown has also been addressed (Davis & Wilcox, 1985; Pulvermuller & Roth, 1991; Leiwo, 1994). Within the social model framework introduced in Chapter 1, these therapies may be viewed as broaching aspects of impairment. An emphasis upon getting the message across – *transaction* – has often been apparent.

While these therapies have proved valuable, they may stop short of promoting communication as a means of *interaction* – that is, as a means of affiliating with others (Simmons-Mackie & Damico, 1995). A focus on communication as a social phenomenon has a number of implications therapeutically: an emphasis upon communication as a collaborative act; the use of 'real-life' encounters to extend communication opportunities; adoption of techniques to optimise communicative access; and the use of conversation as a means of community reintegration (Kagan & Gailey, 1993; Pound, 1996; Lyon *et al*, 1997; Simmons-Mackie, 1998). This approach, explicitly addressing the actions of communication partnerships rather than those of the aphasic person alone, may therefore be used to reduce the disabling consequences of aphasia.

At the aphasia centre, our therapies borrow from both of these traditions. While we endeavour to minimise the communicative burden and isolation experienced by people with aphasia (for example, by training relatives and others to be skilled conversation partners), we also recognise that our clients operate in a wider world, one that is generally aphasia-unfriendly. Certain of our therapy programmes, therefore, aim directly to improve the client's communicative effectiveness. The therapies outlined in this chapter address Total Communication, communicative drawing and the use of communication books. In the final section of the chapter, we describe therapies that focus on conversation and the attempt to create richer communication environments for our clients.

Working on communication and conversation in groups

Many of the therapy ideas presented in this chapter can be adapted for use with individuals or in group sessions. In Chapter 2, we outlined some of the benefits of groupwork. Groups provide an ideal environment for the introduction of communication techniques; multiple chances for observing and practising strategies occur, along with peer feedback and reinforcement. They are also useful as a forum for discussion, disclosure and support. Perhaps more importantly, groups provide their members with opportunities for true communicative and conversational encounters. In this sense, groups may play a role in helping to transfer clinical skills to more everyday contexts.

Family involvement in communication and conversation

It almost goes without saying that family members can also play a key role in facilitating the client's acquisition of new techniques. They can create opportunities for strategies to be practised and used, and are an important source of encouragement. Of course, they themselves need assistance to do this. We find that family members benefit from explanations of the rationale underlying therapy, opportunities to see techniques being modelled, and practice in supporting the client's use of new methods. They often need help to modify aspects of their own communication, particularly as their aphasic partner's communicative attempts may well be slower, less efficient and more ambiguous than before the onset of aphasia.

In an ideal world, family members would become involved at an early stage and then become regular participants in intervention. In reality, however, the demands faced by families can mean that their involvement is sporadic or brief. We feel it is important to be sensitive to the pressures faced and to be as flexible as possible in our approach. At the aphasia centre we hold regular open days, during which families explore issues related to their relative's aphasia. Where appropriate, home visits are arranged to evaluate and enhance everyday interactions. Video recordings can be used to demonstrate techniques to family members who find it difficult to participate at home or at the centre. Information sheets and regular telephone contact may also support changes in communication and conversation.

Total Communication

Total Communication (Green, 1982; Fawcus *et al*, 1990; Lawson & Fawcus, 1999) refers to an approach, widely used at the aphasia centre, in which clients are encouraged to communicate in any way available to them. When skilfully applied, Total Communication involves flexible use of a number of modalities including speech, gesture, drawing, writing, facial expression and the use of communication books, maps and other environmental 'props'. Of course, mere encouragement to use Total Communication is usually not enough. Clients need practice in using methods and modalities of communication that may, at first, seem alien.

While Total Communication can greatly enhance both transaction and interaction, not all clients can make use of the technique. Strong candidates include those clients who have little or no speech, who seem aware of the impact of their aphasia on communication and who are attempting to use alternative modalities. Clients who appear to do less well include those with limited insight into the nature and effect of their aphasia, and those who are reluctant to use means of communication other than speech.

Introducing Total Communication

We use a diagram to introduce Total Communication to our clients (*see* Figure 3.1). The diagram not only shows different means of communication which may be available to clients, but also acknowledges (through the 'lightbulb' icon) that people with aphasia still have valid thoughts and concepts. The focus of therapy then falls upon revealing these ideas through a variety of communicative methods.

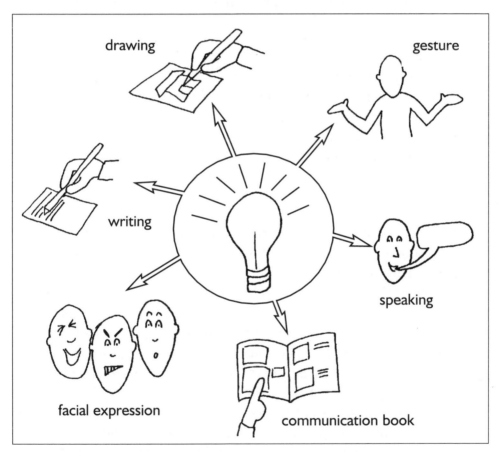

drawing

gesture

writing

speaking

facial expression

communication book

Figure 3.1 *Total Communication*

The diagram can either be presented and explained as it is, or constructed by clients and therapist in an interactive process. This can be done by:

- 'Brainstorming' the communicative modalities that group members currently use.
- Therapist-led role plays demonstrating different methods of communication.
- Watching a video of a group of people with aphasia and noting down the strategies used.
- Viewing snippets of a silent movie (such as Buster Keaton or Mr Bean), again noting down the means of communication used.

Of course, aphasia may affect clients' ability to give information about their own communication, or what they have seen others use. Checklists such as the one in Figure 3.2 can be useful here. The components of the Total Communication diagram (that is, the pictures representing speech, drawing, gesture and so on) can also be presented on separate cards. Clients can then be encouraged to select from these to build up personal communication profiles (for example, to show how they communicate at present) or to describe the modalities they have observed on video or in a group interaction.

Promoting Total Communication in clinical settings

Once introduced to Total Communication, clients need to be supported in its use. This support may take the form of specific activities which prompt the technique and a number of these are outlined below. As valuably, environmental supports may be offered: therapists should be willing to use Total Communication themselves and provide suitable materials and resources for clients' use (pen and paper, maps, timetables and so on). In group settings, care must be taken to create equal access to 'the floor', particularly if some group members can speak and others cannot. The therapist should try to ensure that all group members are given opportunities to participate. The therapist should also accept, reinforce and model non-speech contributions, promoting the idea that 'anything goes' so far as Total Communication is concerned.

Implementing Total Communication

A number of therapeutic activities can be used to implement Total Communication. Broadly speaking, these can be grouped as:

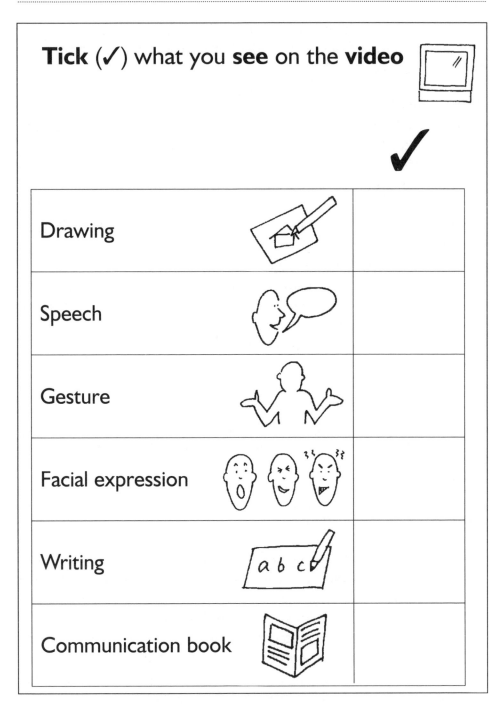

Tick (✓) what you see on the video

Drawing		
Speech		
Gesture		
Facial expression		
Writing		
Communication book		

Figure 3.2 *Observing Total Communication – a checklist*

- Tasks in which the primary emphasis is communication.
- Tasks requiring generation of ideas as well as communication.
- Analytic tasks.

Communication

A variety of PACE-type activities (Davis & Wilcox, 1985) can be used to establish Total Communication. The basic format, in which a client is given a message to communicate to a partner, can be adapted for individual or group sessions. These activities may initially encourage communication via any means, which the therapist will suggest if necessary – for example: 'Can you show me what you do with it?'; 'Can you draw it?'.

Different types of messages will place differing demands on communicative ability, ranging from descriptions of single objects to explanations of everyday events. It is important to consider how the client will receive the original message unambiguously (will it be written, drawn or whispered?), without creating bias toward a particular modality. Mere copying of the message should be discouraged. In group sessions, clients can take turns presenting their messages to each other. Such sessions carry the benefit of peer feedback regarding the intelligibility (or otherwise) of the communication attempt. Some thought needs to be given to how this feedback will be given: the other group members might be given a list of potential messages, from which they choose the one transmitted.

As clients become more skilled, they may be asked to use more than one way of conveying a certain message. This can be important in developing a flexibility of approach:

1 A message is placed in the middle of the table for all group members to see. Group members take it in turns to communicate the message in different ways. Thus the first person may draw the message, the second write it, the third gesture it and so on.
2 Two piles of cards are placed face down in front of group members. One pile contains messages to be communicated; the other, pictures representing various methods of communication. Group members take it in turn to draw one card from each pile, conveying the selected message in the specified manner.

Generation and communication

The use of Total Communication in daily interactions not only requires the application of communicative techniques, but the generation of ideas to power this communication. Tasks may be introduced in the clinical setting to link these two processes. These tasks may initially have little 'real-life' connection; however, it is ultimately useful to move on to activities in which clients explore communicative solutions to everyday situations. For example, clients may use Total Communication to:

- Express personal preferences eg, favourite food, drink, sport, means of relaxation.
- Brainstorm items within a category eg, tools, transport, furniture.
- Add information to a story sequence eg, 'What happens next ...?'
- Outline steps in a common task eg, wrapping a gift, making a cup of tea
- Explain a routine eg, travelling to the aphasia centre, the timetable at a day centre.
- Role play communicative responses to everyday events eg, ordering lunch, asking for directions.

Again, to promote flexible use of communication strategies, clients may be asked to consider alternative ways of getting their message across. Initially, this may be fostered during group feedback. For example, group members may be asked to reflect the message using another modality (for example, gesturing back a message that has been conveyed in writing). In 'brainstorm'-type activities, each group member may be encouraged to use a different method of communication when his or her turn to contribute arises.

Analytic tasks

Skilled and flexible use of Total Communication can also be encouraged through activities encouraging introspection. Clients who are facilitated to explore their communicative strengths are, in our experience, more likely to use them when the need arises and to use suitable back-up methods when a favoured strategy fails. The activities already described in the section 'Introducing Total Communication' can also be used to introduce clients to the idea of monitoring and analysing communication. Other tasks that facilitate introspection include:

- A client is given a message to communicate. Once this is done, the client is asked to identify the modality used by pointing to it on the Total Communication diagram (*see* Figure 3.1). Alternatively, other group members may provide this feedback.
- A group member selects a message to communicate, then, using a rating scale, indicates how effective the modality was in conveying the message. Other group members may be called upon to rate the effectiveness of the modality used. Over time, this method can be used to identify a hierarchy of useful strategies for each client.

There is no doubt, however, that monitoring and evaluating communication can be difficult for people with aphasia. When working in a group, it may be useful to start with tasks in which the whole group makes a judgement on (say) the effectiveness of a modality just witnessed. As the ability to introspect and analyse develops, the group may be divided into smaller units to complete certain activities. For example, two clients may work together to watch a role play and then complete a checklist about the communication strategies observed.

Moving Total Communication into the everyday environment
The procedures described above crucially support the next stage of therapy, in which Total Communication skills are transferred to more everyday environments. We have found that different groups and individuals move through the elements of Total Communication therapy at different speeds. Some spend considerable time in the initial stages, exploring what Total Communication is and gaining practice in conveying messages. Others quickly move on to analytic tasks and begin to explore issues in transfer. Table 3.1 charts the progress of one group who had already had some exposure to Total Communication techniques.

Moving Total Communication out of the centre and into everyday life provides a challenge to client and therapist alike. *When* this transfer of ability can be facilitated, and *how advanced* Total Communication skills need to be before transfer can occur, will depend upon the type of environment the client is trying to access. We feel that therapy within the home can begin soon after Total Communication is introduced. Family members may work with client and therapist to create an environment

Table 3.1 *One group's progress through Total Communication therapy*

	Overall therapy theme(s)	Example methods
Weeks 1–4	Introduction to Total Communication Generation and communication	• Detailed introduction to Total Communication at start of each session – including explanation of TC diagram, reflection upon modalities already used by group members, discussion of when TC might be useful (eg, generally, in communication, as well as in repair) • Divergent semantic task (eg, making a list of items that might be taken on a trip to the Amazon) in which group members are encouraged to use any available modality • Therapist-led feedback regarding TC modalities used in task, including identification of strategies used by particular group members
Weeks 5–10	Analytic tasks	• Regular whole group 'brainstorm' of components of TC diagram • One client is given the name of an object/event to communicate to the group. This name is made known to all to assist a focus upon *how* the message is conveyed. The other group members use the TC diagram to pinpoint the modality used • As for task above, but with individual clients identifying the modality *they* used when communicating the message • A client is given a composite picture (eg, a kitchen scene), and asked to select one item to communicate. The other group members indicate (a) the modality used, and (b) an alternative way in which the message could be conveyed • Divergent semantic tasks (eg, what would you be doing if you weren't at the aphasia centre?), with whole group reflection upon modalities employed
Weeks 11–13	Transfer of skill	• Identification, by group members, of situations where TC could be used effectively • Role play of specific communication situations (eg, asking for an item at a shop; explaining symptoms to a doctor) • Each group member is given a message to communicate to his or her spouse. The spouse completes a feedback form, indicating which components of the message were received and how this information was conveyed

that supports acquisition and use of the technique. Use of Total Communication in public places, such as shops and restaurants, may require more developed and robust abilities, largely because the presence of skilled communication partners cannot be guaranteed.

Working with families
While some families readily grasp the rationale behind Total Communication and are eager to support it, others may find the concept difficult or alien. Most people benefit from some preliminary discussion regarding the nature of their relative's aphasia and why Total Communication may be useful. These discussions should involve consideration of the clients' communicative strengths. In some instances, it may be appropriate to ask family members to collect evidence regarding current means of communication. They can do this by:

- Completing a profile of communicative function (for example, the Pragmatics Profile of Everyday Communication Skills in Adults [Dewart & Summers, 1996]).
- Keeping a daily diary in which specific examples of (say) non-speech communication are recorded.
- Completing a checklist regarding the communication strategies used in a designated situation (for example, having a conversation with the grandchildren).

Families can also benefit from seeing techniques modelled and reinforced. They may watch individual or group sessions, or a conversation between client and therapist, in which Total Communication is used. It can be useful to offer some structure for family members' observations. For example, they could be asked to complete a short questionnaire on the communication strategies used, or comment on what the therapist did to encourage Total Communication.

The insights provided by this process of structured observation and reflection can assist the next stage of therapy, in which families begin to support the client's use of Total Communication more directly. Almost inevitably, family members need to modify aspects of their own communication in order to interpret the client's attempts appropriately.

This can be done in a number of ways:

- Family members take part in a role play in which the therapist uses Total Communication. The therapist provides feedback on what was useful (or otherwise) in the family's attempts to facilitate Total Communication.
- Family members (and therapist) watch a video of one of their own interactions with the person who has aphasia. After the video, they discuss features of their communication that helped and hindered the person's use of Total Communication.

Once identified, changes to family members' communication can be facilitated through a modified version of Conversational Coaching (Holland, 1991). This technique is ordinarily used to assist people with aphasia in developing their communicative and conversational skills. A typical task involves the client being asked to convey a message that is a little in advance of his or her communicative ability. Client and therapist discuss and practise different means of getting the message across; the client then uses the agreed method to communicate the message to another person. 'On-line' coaching may also occur: that is, the therapist may intervene, during the communication attempt, to suggest alternative methods. In the case of family members, Conversational Coaching may be used (for example) to explore ways of framing questions so that they can be answered via drawing or gesture, or to develop techniques for conversational repair. Families can also be encouraged to allow extra time for communication to occur and to use Total Communication to verify any messages received.

Communicating in everyday environments
As noted before, using Total Communication in other environments probably demands more robust skills. Transfer of Total Communication strategies may be helped if client and therapist spend some time identifying regularly occurring communicative situations, and habitual communication partners. If possible, the types of messages transmitted should also be discussed (*see* Figure 3.3).

A hierarchy of communication situations can then be developed with the intention of first using Total Communication in situations deemed

	MONDAY	TUESDAY	WEDNESDAY	THURSDAY	FRIDAY	SATURDAY	SUNDAY
A C T I V I T Y	1 Aphasia Centre	1 Day Centre	1 Day Centre	1 Speech & Language Therapy	1 Aphasia Centre	1 Watch TV	1 Watch TV
	2 Home	2 Home	2 Home	2 Home	2 Home	2 Family visit	2 Family visit
						3 Pub	3 Pub
P A R T N E R	1 • Staff • Students • Group members • Taxi driver	1 • Staff • Group members		1 Speech & Language Therapist	1 • Staff • Students • Group members • Taxi driver	1 Wife	
	2 Family	2 Family	2 Family	2 Family	2 Family	2 Daughter	
						3 • Bar staff • Neighbours	

Figure 3.3 *A profile of everyday communication*

less demanding. Role play can be invaluable in exploring different ways of communicating in each situation. The client may also wish to develop some material that explains aphasia and Total Communication, for use with partners who are unfamiliar with these terms. Repeated exposure to the same situation (for example, communicating in the Post Office) can assist the client in identifying a core set of useful strategies.

Transitional work of this kind can also be carried out in groups. Group therapy carries the advantage of extra heads to reflect, discuss and brainstorm creative solutions to everyday problems, as well as providing moral support. Clients may also feel more comfortable using Total Communication in outside environments when supported by their peers.

Case Study 3.1 Total Communication: the pub outing

The group involved in this therapy programme comprises between six and eight people with severe aphasia who are facilitated by a speech and language therapist and four student therapists. While there is some variation in their language and communication skills, most group members have impaired auditory comprehension and little or no speech. Most have significant difficulty understanding single written words and few can write anything other than their own name.

Despite these restrictions, all group members retain some means of effective communication, typically facial expression and/ or natural gesture. Other ways of interacting (for example, drawing or the use of a communication book) may have developed in response to therapy. The group therapy aims to maximise these skills, and a philosophy of Total Communication is adopted. As well as promoting communicative ability, therapy may address topics such as stress management and conversation skills.

While much of this therapy happens within the aphasia centre, frequent attempts are made to transfer skills to everyday settings. Relatives are encouraged to attend sessions in order to develop individually tailored communication strategies. Home visits are made to observe and discuss features of the communicative environment and to set relevant goals. Group therapy programmes have been devised to provide opportunities for clients to develop and practise strategies for dealing with communicative situations outside the home. These have also proved useful in providing a forum for clients to address barriers to daily communication.

Moving Total Communication outside

A recent therapy programme has involved group members preparing for and participating in an end-of-year outing to a local pub. A pub trip was unanimously selected by the group members because it would be enjoyable, and because it would also provide a number of communication opportunities (for example, ordering drinks and food). Several group members indicated they had not been to the pub since their stroke, partly because of communication difficulties. Some did go to their local, but relied on others to communicate for them when they were there.

An 11-week programme of therapy based around the pub trip was devised. Early on, group members were encouraged to reflect upon the therapeutic benefits of going to the pub. Members who struggled to generate their own ideas were given a set of cue cards, some depicting valid benefits and others 'red herrings', from which they were encouraged to choose. The following goals were set by the student speech and language therapists facilitating the group:

- Group members will use Total Communication in all stages of planning the group outing.
- Group members will use Total Communication strategies outside the centre to carry out everyday tasks.
- Group members will use Total Communication when interacting with each other in a social context.
- Group members will demonstrate their confidence in Total Communication by using it with strangers.

In Week 2, a brief trip was made to the pub to identify the communication situations in which group members would be involved. As well as the obvious situations, members identified communication opportunities such as asking for the juke-box to be turned on and asking where the toilet was. Using Total Communication, group members also identified *barriers* that might lead to their exclusion from the pub and similar social opportunities in everyday life. These barriers included:

- Pub too far away to walk and no suitable transport.
- Restricted access to the pub for wheelchair users (mainly in the form of steps into and within the pub).
- Inaccessible toilets.
- Expensive food and drinks.

The group subsequently decided they would only go on the outing if an accessible pub could be found. In Week 3, the session was devoted to brainstorming a set of access criteria. An appraisal form (see Figure 3.4) was developed for use during the group's visits to other pubs in Weeks 4 and 5; some members used these sessions to gain extra experience in ordering drinks!

Once an accessible pub was found, group members engaged in a number of tasks designed to address the use of Total Communication strategies. The communication opportunities and potential barriers which might arise were systematically reviewed. Group members were encouraged to demonstrate their responses to these using role play (for example, using a communication book to order a beer, or gesture to show that a meal had gone cold). In one session, the group addressed potential barriers to whole group conversations in the pub environment (for example, loud music). Solutions to these problems were discussed (asking a barperson to turn the music down; moving seats closer) and Total Communication strategies were selected.

An important part of the planning was the identification and evaluation of individual goals for involvement in the outing. These were set in the week before the end-of-year trip and reflected the previous weeks' discussions. Group members were encouraged to describe their personal goals in any way possible and one example of this is shown in Figure 3.5. All group members' goals were evaluated in Week 11, after the outing.

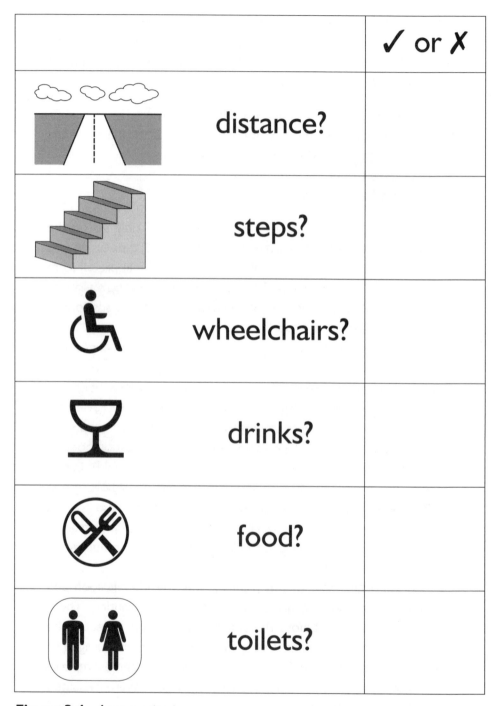

	✓ or ✗
distance?	
steps?	
wheelchairs?	
drinks?	
food?	
toilets?	

Figure 3.4 *Access criteria*

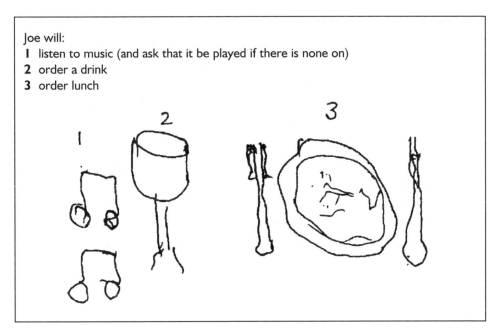

Joe will:
1 listen to music (and ask that it be played if there is none on)
2 order a drink
3 order lunch

Figure 3.5 *Individual goals for the pub trip*

Evaluation
After the trip, a review of individual goals revealed that all group members met their criteria for involvement. Reviewing the therapy goals, the student therapists found that members used Total Communication in planning the trip, and without hesitation when ordering food and drink at the pub. They also used a variety of communication strategies when conversing with each other. In overall appraisal of the therapy programme, the students attributed their success to:

- Group members' active involvement in planning the trip and in identifying communicative opportunities and barriers
- Sufficient opportunity for group members to practise relevant Total Communication strategies.
- The process of setting and completing individual goals.

Group members were also encouraged to set a goal for a future trip to the pub with family or friends. At this stage, it became apparent that while certain group members had enjoyed the therapy-focused outing, it was unlikely they would visit their local. The three group members who still went to the pub agreed that, on their next visit, they would order their own drinks using Total Communication. Their partners were informed of this goal.

In effect, although they visited the pub several times subsequently, these group members did not order drinks independently. This was either because their partners did the ordering automatically, or because it was easier not to embark upon Total Communication. This finding raises some complex issues regarding independence or autonomy as a therapeutic goal, and the potential barriers raised, however unwittingly, by family and friends. Exploration of habitual communication roles, and identification of situations in which both client and family are happy for Total Communication to proceed, may be important in establishing the technique.

Communicative drawing

There is a growing literature regarding the use of communicative drawing by people with aphasia (for example, Trupe, 1986; Lyon & Helm-Estabrooks, 1987; Lyon & Sims, 1989; Lyon, 1995; Sacchett et al, 1999). This literature reflects our own observations that some people, despite markedly impaired language, have drawing skills which are relatively preserved or are amenable to therapy. Drawing is also attractive, communicatively and therapeutically, because it provides a fixed record of an exchange. This can be accepted, modified or elaborated as the interactants see fit, or form the basis for discussion and analysis in more therapeutic settings. Drawing, therefore, has several benefits that do not accompany other, more transient forms of communication (for example, speech and gesture).

Lyon (1995) notes that two distinctive approaches to drawing therapy exist. The first, motivated by the premise that drawing may act as a substitute for language, focuses on the production of recognisable drawings. Therapy tasks are devised to increase the accuracy of the client's drawings, with the aim of promoting communicative independence. The second approach views drawing as an augmentative form of communication, in which it complements rather than replaces language. A focus upon interpersonal aspects of communication characterises this approach. Correspondingly, communication is seen to be the responsibility of all communication partners and the training of non-aphasic people in facilitative strategies is an integral part of therapy.

In a number of ways, the differences between these two approaches to drawing mirror the differences that underlie therapies addressing transaction and interaction. As in the case of these latter therapies, our approach to communicative drawing is to take the middle ground: the interventions outlined in this section variously address the skills of the person with aphasia and the communicative partnership, in order to enhance communication and conversation in a range of contexts.

While drawing can be an extremely useful means of communication, it is important to recognise that some people with aphasia will have considerable difficulty in using this modality. Central processing, visuoconstructional and motor execution impairments may well interfere with a person's ability to draw (Gainotti et al, 1983; Kirk & Kertesz, 1989; Lyon, 1995). Lyon (1995) also notes that clients may well be less likely to use drawing if they are able to summon quicker and more conventional means of communication such as speech, gesture or writing. Although we share this view, we have also worked with several more verbal clients who employ drawing when other forms of communication fail.

Drawings produced by people with aphasia are typically reduced in detail. Some difficulty in dealing with perspective may also be apparent, and drawings can be small and difficult to make out (Lyon, 1995; Sacchett et al, 1999). Experience of drawing prior to the onset of aphasia can also influence the planning of therapy; clients may feel embarrassed and reluctant to draw and this needs to be acknowledged and addressed before therapy can proceed. The next section offers some ideas for introducing communicative drawing and promoting generative drawing. We go on to describe activities that focus on the use of appropriate size and level of detail within communicative drawings.

Introducing communicative drawing

When introducing communicative drawing, the therapist aims to present it as a viable form of communication and attempts to overcome any reluctance to use this modality. To this end, it may be valuable to begin therapy with discussion of how drawing is used in everyday contexts. Clients may be facilitated to brainstorm situations in which they might see drawings or diagrams (for example, when travelling on the Underground). Alternatively, drawings from other mainstream sources may be presented (for example, political sketches, cartoons, diagrams from instruction manuals), with some exploration of their meaning. The therapist's own use of communicative drawing may help the client to feel more confident and to accept the technique.

As with the tasks used to introduce Total Communication, PACE-like activities (Davis & Wilcox, 1985) may also be used to introduce communicative drawing. Clients may be provided with information about everyday objects to convey to a partner via drawing. Again, some thought should be given to how this information will be communicated to the drawer. Picture stimuli should be used sparingly, to discourage clients from simply copying what they see rather than producing their own representations. The complexity of this kind of task may be varied by introducing less common objects or simple events as stimuli. Another way of introducing drawing is to provide clients with a basic shape and ask them to add sufficient detail to transform the shape to represent a specified object. This task can be particularly useful for clients whose skills are not sufficient to support function in PACE-type activities.

Generative drawing

Drawing in response to a given stimulus is very different from drawing in a communicative setting, not least because communicative drawing requires the generation of ideas and concepts before pen is put to paper (Sacchett *et al*, 1999). Some activities encouraging the linking of ideas and communication have already been mentioned in the description of Total Communication therapy. Sacchett *et al* outline other tasks that are useful in establishing generative drawing:

Drawing absent objects
- Immediate recall (eg, Kim's Game)
- Semantically cued objects (eg, things that go together; complete the category)

Generating information around a theme
- Things that go with … (eg, sports equipment; tools of trade)
- Things you find in … (eg, bathroom, fridge, garden shed)
- Things you need for … (eg, putting up shelves; making a cup of tea; baking a cake)

While the above tasks are designed to prompt object-based drawings, they may be modified to elicit the drawing of events. Clients may be presented with a sequence of action pictures and asked to draw 'what happens next'. Themed, event-based drawings may be produced in response to requests to draw (say) things that people do on holiday or in their spare time, hated chores or bad habits.

In addition to working with clients to develop their ability to summon up and execute representations, it can be useful to address more general skills to support communication. Therapy may aim to improve the client's ability to attend and respond to the communication partner. Client and therapist may also discuss strategies to assist partners' understanding of drawn messages. This may include conveying one piece of information at a time, adding detail to misunderstood attempts and supplementing drawing with Total Communication where necessary. We would suggest that these issues are tackled early on. Such an approach, which explicitly recognises and explores the needs of others, is important in the transfer of skills to more everyday environments.

Refining drawing skills

Of the therapies outlined here, those attempting to refine the quality of the client's drawing are likely to prove contentious. As noted previously, while some therapy approaches directly address drawing accuracy, others see communicative drawing as the responsibility of the communication partnership (Lyon, 1995). In this latter approach, drawing clarity and accuracy are not prerequisites for its use. Rather, therapy involves training non-aphasic people to facilitate the drawn communication of their aphasic partners. While we support this approach, we also recognise that people with aphasia may need to communicate with others who are unused to communicative drawing, or have limited facilitation skills. For this reason, we often work with clients on improving the quality of their drawings, paying particular attention to size and level of detail.

Therapy to promote appropriate size and detail in drawing
Therapies to promote appropriately sized drawings can be relatively straightforward. Clients can be encouraged to produce only one drawing per page, and to make that drawing as big as possible. The therapeutic strategy of enlargement can also be used (Lyon, 1995) (*see also* 'Using facilitative techniques', later in this chapter). Therapies addressing detail are a little more complicated and will depend upon whether the client is producing too much or too little detail in their drawings.

Too much detail

1   Each group member is given his or her own photograph of a very detailed object or scene (for example, a vase with an intricate design; a person wearing highly patterned clothes) and asked to point to the features that would be minimally included in a communicative drawing of the item. The group member draws these minimal features onto a separate piece of paper. This drawing is then shown to the rest of the group; group members are asked to identify the object by selecting its name from a (pre-prepared) list of options.

2   Clients work in pairs, taking turns to select a card from a pile placed face down on the table. When a client selects a card, he or she is asked to draw the item or event written on the card. The partner is instructed to interrupt him as soon as the drawing is detailed enough to be understood.

Too little detail

1   Each group member is given a card, upon which is written the name of an object. The objects to be drawn comprise the same basic shape – for example, they may be all round (a pound coin, the sun, a ring) or all rectangular (a ladder, a ruler, a pencil). Group members are given a few minutes to draw their item; each then shows his or her drawing to the group in turn. The others feed back their understanding of the item by pointing to its name on a list. If they are unable to identify the object, or indicate another (similarly shaped) item on the list, the group member who prepared the drawing is asked to add more detail.

2   One group member is asked to generate and draw an item conforming to a specified shape (for example, round, square, rectangular). Others in the group use Total Communication to convey their understanding of the drawn item, with the original group member adding detail as necessary. Group members then take turns to generate and draw different objects that share the same basic shape.

Monitoring tasks

Monitoring tasks can also enable consistent consideration of size and detail and can effect changes in drawing clarity. An ability to judge the adequacy of one's own drawings is important in communicative repair. As size and detail are abstract concepts, it may be useful to represent them using pictures (*see* Figure 3.6). Alternative ways of referring to size and detail can also help understanding of what is required. Some clients respond more readily when asked if a drawing is 'big enough' or if it has all of the 'important parts'.

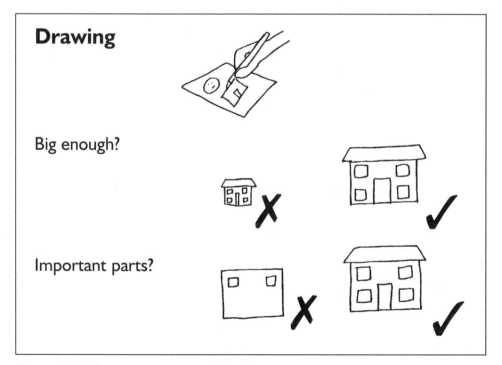

Figure 3.6 *Drawing on size and detail*

Some clients find it easier to appraise others' drawings before considering their own. The following tasks can facilitate clients' monitoring of size and detail:

- The client sorts examples of the therapist's drawings into piles marked 'clear' and 'not clear'.
- The client sorts the drawings that are 'not clear' according to whether the problem concerns size or detail.
- The client uses a scale to rate the achievement of appropriate size and/or level of detail in their own and other peoples' communicative drawings.
- The therapist establishes routine appraisal by clients of their communicative drawing: Is it big enough? Does it have all the important parts?
- Using clear drawings as exemplars, the therapist encourages identification of details that helped clients' recognition.

Communicative drawing in everyday contexts: towards interactive drawing

We feel that people with aphasia are unlikely to use communicative drawing in everyday contexts without direct support and encouragement. Of course, this difficulty is not unique to drawing, but the fact that drawing is seldom used in ordinary communication can make it difficult to establish. As with Total Communication, clients may benefit from constructing and working through a hierarchy of communication situations when first using drawing in everyday environments.

In addition, non-aphasic partners often need specific training in how to facilitate drawing in order to optimise communication attempts. In the remainder of this section, we will therefore focus on therapies suitable for family members or other regular communication partners. In creating a facilitative environment, and with attention to factors that create the 'feel and flow' of natural conversation (Kagan & Gailey, 1993) (*see also* the section 'Conversationally-based therapies' later in this chapter) family members may help to bridge the gap between drawing being used as a communicative tool and it being used interactively.

Working with family members

As with Total Communication, family members are likely to benefit from discussing the rationale of communicative drawing and seeing it in action. Activities used to introduce communicative drawing to people with aphasia can also be used with their communicative partners. Early on, it is often useful to ask family members to participate in PACE-type activities during which they have a chance to do some drawing themselves. This kind of task can be useful in revealing that messages can be conveyed via drawing. It can also offer some useful insights into how the family can make drawing more accessible and acceptable. Other tasks relate to exploring and utilising facilitative techniques.

Exploring facilitative techniques

1   Family members watch a video of the person with aphasia using communicative drawings with the therapist. They note down: (a) what sorts of messages were conveyed and (b) strategies used by the therapist to facilitate communicative drawing. They may use a checklist to guide their observations.

2   Family members watch a video of their own interactions with the person who has aphasia. They are encouraged to discuss when drawing could have been used in the interaction and how they would have encouraged their relative to draw.

The following list, adapted from a case study of communicative drawing, illustrates several facilitative strategies that family members might use (Sacchett & Lindsay, 1998).

- Ask 'homing-in' questions (yes/no type) about the drawing before trying to guess what it is.
- Ask your partner to show you the important parts of the drawing, and then to draw them again bigger if you do not recognise them.
- Ask your partner for other clues: 'Show me what you do with it.' 'Show me how big it is.'
- Add to, or change, your partner's drawing by drawing something yourself: your 'best guess'.
- Write down key words about the drawing as you find things out.

Using facilitative techniques

Once identified, facilitative techniques can be systematically practised and reinforced in therapy with family members. Where a number of potential strategies have been identified, it may be useful initially to choose one or two that family members feel confident in using. A select set of strategies consistently used are generally more facilitative than a larger number used sporadically. Therapy along the lines of Conversational Coaching (Holland, 1991) can be useful. Techniques can also be 'tried out' with the therapist before they are used with the person who has aphasia.

One useful technique is *enlargement* (Lyon, 1995). We have found that this technique is particularly applicable to drawings that are difficult to understand because they comprise a number of small components or they contain superfluous detail. Enlargement involves asking the client to point to the most important part of the drawing and then to produce a bigger drawing of just that part. Other strategies include asking the person with aphasia to add details to their drawings, to depict changes over time using a sequence of drawings, and to indicate which 'view' has been portrayed (for example, the side view or the view from above [Lyon, 1995]).

Case Study 3.2 Using communicative drawing: Janet's story

Janet, who is 69, joined the aphasia centre 18 months after she had a stroke which left her with severe aphasia. Prior to her stroke, Janet had enjoyed an active retirement with her husband, Derek. Her interests included reading, gardening and sewing and she had been a regular churchgoer. Janet had three months' intensive rehabilitation and then weekly outpatient speech and language therapy. Her therapy had largely focused upon aspects of her language impairment including central semantic processing and her use of the phonological output lexicon. Janet had spontaneously used drawing to communicate in some therapy sessions, but this skill remained relatively unexplored.

Initial assessment at the aphasia centre showed that, while her auditory comprehension was reasonably intact, Janet's spoken output was restricted to 'yes' and 'no'. Her reading and writing were impaired at the single-word level. Janet's communication proceeded through facial expression and natural gesture and she used pictographs provided by her therapist. She had a communication book, containing information about objects and events, but did not use it. Evaluation of her drawing skills showed an ability to draw several common objects on request and to provide a sketch showing an aerial view of her house and garden. She could also draw some items within a designated category. Janet's drawings varied in clarity and were sometimes over-elaborate (see Figure 3.7).

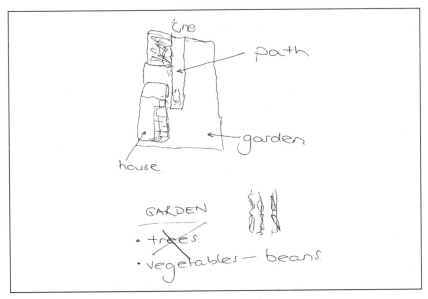

Figure 3.7 *Janet: drawings produced during initial assessment*

Following further assessment, Janet joined a group of people who had similar levels of impairment. Together, she and the therapist negotiated that they would work primarily on non-verbal methods of communication. It was agreed that individual sessions would initially be devoted to refining and personalising Janet's communication book, while communicative drawing would be addressed within the group itself.

Drawing therapy
Janet took part in a group-based programme of drawing therapy. This consisted of 14 sessions lasting about 45 minutes, which took place over a period of 18 weeks. The following goals were specified:

- Group members will exchange information about everyday items and scenarios through drawing.
- Group members will produce drawings that are sufficiently large and detailed enough to be interpreted by others.
- They will aim to provide accurate feedback on the adequacy of their own and others' communicative drawings.

Two of the group members had never drawn communicatively before, so the first three weeks of therapy introduced the technique and generated basic communication through the use of PACE-type activities. Monitoring tasks were gradually introduced. Group members were shown photographs of objects that included both necessary and superfluous detail. They were encouraged to indicate which features would be included in a communicative drawing of the object. They were also shown 'inadequate' drawings prepared by the student therapists and were asked to indicate in each case whether the size or the detail was causing problems of interpretation. They then moved on to producing drawings themselves, for example, taking a card with an object written on it, drawing the object and showing other members of the group. Group feedback was encouraged.

As group members became more able to analyse and produce simple communicative drawings, activities prompting the inclusion of contextual cues were introduced. Thus, group members were asked to think of a prized possession at home, to draw it, and to indicate its location by drawing at least one other item in the same room. The other group members had to guess the item and its location (using a list of rooms as a prompt).

Another activity involved group members working on two scenarios involving the same object or person in different locations (for example, a woman going to church and a woman going to the shops). They were asked to draw both scenarios and to include appropriate information regarding place. The pictures were then shown to the other group members, who were encouraged to identify the location specified in each picture.

Janet proved to be an active and able participant in this therapy. She drew readily, and made accurate judgements about the size and detail of others' communicative drawings. She also modified her own drawings in the light of others' feedback. Her drawings increased in clarity (see Figure 3.8) and she began to use them communicatively (see Figure 3.9).

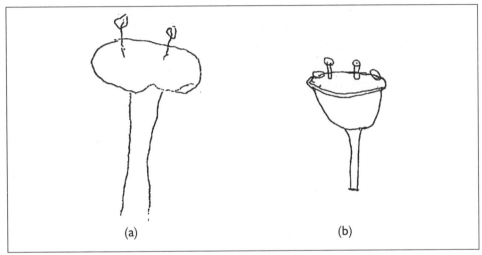

(a)   (b)

Figure 3.8 *Janet: a comparison of drawings (of a washbasin) made in (a) Week 1 and (b) Week 14*

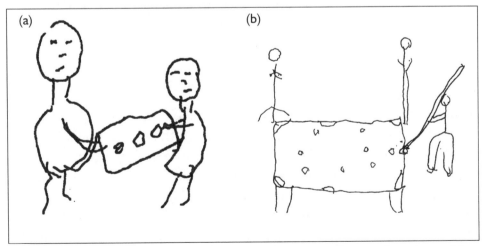

(a)   (b)

Figure 3.9 *Janet: current drawing skills (a) Janet explaining that she and her husband play board games, (b) Janet explaining that she likes to watch snooker.*

Transferring skills to everyday environments

During this period of therapy, Janet's husband began to meet with her student keyworker in order to develop skills in facilitating non-verbal communication. Several sessions were spent exploring the impact of aphasia upon everyday interactions and the rationale for using non-verbal modalities. Derek observed group therapy sessions and watched videotapes of him and Janet conversing. He was encouraged to think about practical ways of supporting Janet's communication beyond the centre.

While he acknowledged Janet's ability to use communicative drawing, Derek was rather unenthusiastic about this modality. He felt that it was too slow for everyday communication and would interfere with their routine. He could not identify a situation in which drawing could be used. He also felt uncertain about his own interpretation skills and declined the offer to address these in therapy. Derek has chosen instead to work with Janet in developing and using her communication book. Nevertheless, Derek encourages Janet to use drawing with friends and ensures she has pen and paper with her when she goes out. Janet continues to work on using drawing with others, and is particularly keen to combine drawing and her residual writing skills in correspondence (for example, to send greeting cards). She also plans to devise a leaflet that explains communicative drawing and includes tips for interpretation.

Communication books

While recent literature is generally positive about the role and benefits of communicative drawing in aphasia therapy (although *see* Cubelli (1995) for an alternative viewpoint), the literature surrounding communication books is more equivocal (Kraat, 1990; Bellaire *et al*, 1991; Blackstone, 1991a; Grist *et al*, 1993; Pyatak Fletcher, 1997). This is disappointing, given that communication books are often introduced early on in rehabilitation, particularly if a client has severe aphasia. It is not unusual for clients to come to the aphasia centre having had at least one communication book devised for them in the past.

Interestingly, few of these clients spontaneously use their books and in this they seem to be typical of others with aphasia. Various reasons for this have been put forward (Kraat, 1990; Pyatak Fletcher, 1997). It is suggested that some people with aphasia lack the necessary linguistic and cognitive skill to use a book successfully. Aphasia itself can disrupt the understanding and use of symbols, and clients may fail to recognise the book's communicative power and potential. Kraat (1990) suggests that there has been some tendency to assign non-speech communication systems to people with aphasia, without proper consideration and appreciation of clients' strengths and existing methods of communication. Insufficiently rigorous selection procedures may, therefore, lie at the heart of some clients' problems with communication books.

Communication books may also remain underused because they contain vocabulary that is of limited relevance or out of date. This may include items that are particularly prone to the influence of aphasia (for example, low imageability words). The vocabulary may also be presented in a relatively inaccessible form. In addition, certain approaches to therapy may limit the use of the book: therapy based on enhancing within-clinic and therapist–client interactions may not expose the potential of a communication book in other contexts. The way in which a communication book and vocabulary are constructed, together with therapeutic methods, can have a profound effect upon the success or otherwise of the endeavour.

While advances in technology have lead to the development of more sophisticated computer-based communication aids (Grist *et al*, 1993; Waller *et al*, 1998), we anticipate that communication books will continue to be tried with aphasic clients. It is for this reason, and because some clients clearly benefit from book use, that communication books are discussed here. We also venture that some key issues in introducing communication books (for example, client skills, selection of a core vocabulary) are broadly similar to those faced when implementing other communication devices with aphasic people.

Considering client skills

It is probably true to say that communication books are often used somewhat haphazardly. Particularly when working with people who have severe aphasia, the attraction of a system entirely composed of pictures rather than words, which can be accessed by an action as simple as pointing, may be great. However, this enthusiasm can oversimplify the intrinsically complex process of communication book use – a process which demands an understanding of symbolic information, the ability to select an item from an array of concepts which are often semantically related, and a recognition of the communicative power that the book can bring. The paring down of an idea, and its representation through an often small set of symbols, is a highly skilled act in itself.

It is also true to say, however, that the skills prerequisite for communication book use remain relatively underexplained. In particular, necessary language skills may be underspecified. It is not surprising then that communication books are sometimes wrongly offered and remain unused. We have found that clients need to have a sufficiently robust semantic system to allow them to select from items grouped within categories, and to derive meaning from pictures and/or photographs at least. Written word-, phrase- or sentence-based books require correspondingly intact reading comprehension. Other requisite abilities include sufficient visual and motoric ability to allow perception and selection of symbols (Beukelman & Mirenda, 1992) and an ability to initiate communication as well as to respond to others.

Clients also need to recognise that items within the book correspond to objects and events in the environment, and can be used to refer to these. Importantly, clients should be able to understand that the book has the power to influence others and get things done. Insights into a client's ability to do this may come through observing daily interactions. Clients who use maps and calendars communicatively, or point to pictures of staff and/or timetables in clinic to get their message across, are likely candidates for communication book use. It is also important to recognise that communication books are not only useful to people with severely impaired language; clients with mild aphasia may use such a book to facilitate communication of proper names, for example (Hux *et al*, 1994).

In addition to client skills, a vital precursor to book use is family and caregiver support for the new system of communication (Blackstone, 1991b; Beukelman & Mirenda, 1992; Hux *et al*, 1994). Their early involvement in devising and implementing the communication book is strongly recommended. Again, aspects of their interactions may need to be modified if the book is to be employed successfully.

Constructing a communication book

Communication books come in a variety of forms, reflecting considerations such as vocabulary size, ease of modification, portability and personal preference. The size of the communication book may be an issue for some clients, particularly if they wish to conceal their aphasia (and need for alternative means of communication) from other people. Table 3.2 describes different forms of communication book commonly used by clients at the aphasia centre and lists their advantages and disadvantages.

Table 3.2 *Advantages and disadvantages of different types of communication books*

Communication book type	Advantages	Disadvantages
Pocket-sized photograph album	Discrete; portable; easily modified	Limited amount of information per page; cannot add extra pages
A4 Photograph album	Easily modified; potentially large amount of information per page	Obvious to others; less portable; cannot add extra pages
A4 Ring binder	Business-like; easily modified; potentially large amount of information per page; can add extra pages	Obvious to others; less portable
Personal organiser	Discrete; business-like; portable; easily modified; can add extra pages	Limited amount of information per page

As the type of communication book selected can influence the number of vocabulary items contained within, it is useful for client and therapist to reach an early decision about the form the book will take. It is also important to give some thought to how information will be presented. Decisions to be made include:

- Written or pictured information? Or a combination of both?
- If written information is used, should this be single words, phrases, sentences, paragraphs?
- If pictures are used: Photographs or drawings? Colour or black and white?
- Number of items per page? Spacing of items?

Some of these decisions may be made on the basis of how the client manages from day to day at the centre. For example, the therapist may be able to estimate reading comprehension abilities quite easily. Other decisions may need to be based on informal assessment; 'mock ups' of communication book pages in different formats may be used to identify accessible graphics and layout.

Other aspects of communication book construction will only become clear when a vocabulary has been selected, including decisions about how information will be categorised, and the order in which these categories will appear. Several authors suggest that a tab system can be used to facilitate clients' access to categorised information (Beukelman *et al*, 1985; Garrett *et al*, 1989). We have used colour-coded pages (that is, one colour per category, and each category a different colour) to the same effect.

Constructing a vocabulary

The issue of vocabulary construction has received much attention (Beukelman & Mirenda, 1992; Hux *et al*, 1994; Pyatak Fletcher, 1997). There is general agreement that items selected should reflect the client's wants and needs, and should allow communication in a variety of everyday settings. Many books contain information about everyday routines (for example, shaving, dressing, washing) and personal possessions (for example, radio, television, toothbrush). However, we agree with Hux *et al* (1994) that such items may actually be used infrequently, primarily because they *are* associated with routines (events that happen regularly, with little variation in how they occur). True communication within these encounters may only arise if something extraordinary takes place. It is also clear that, as they adapt to life post-stroke, family members and caregivers learn to pre-empt their aphasic partner's basic wants and needs. Again, recourse to corresponding items in the communication book may be uncommon. Having said that, the occasional need for reference to wants and needs is sufficient to warrant the inclusion of certain, individually relevant vocabulary items to deal with the unusual. Hux *et al* (1994) warn that therapists must take care to balance this type of information with other items which have different communicative functions.

Three further aspects of communication are suggested for inclusion (Light, 1988). These are:

- Communication to share information.
- Communication to foster social closeness.
- Communication to comply with rules of social etiquette.

The ability to *share information* is vitally important. Our clients often request that names of family members, friends, favourite pastimes and commonly visited places are included in their books for just this purpose. The transmission of truly novel messages is more of a challenge, perhaps requiring concepts and vocabulary that do not appear within the communication book. In order to facilitate communication of new information, we encourage clients to collect relevant material (for example, newspaper articles, photographs, football programmes) to keep in a pocket or envelope within their book. This can then be used to initiate or support communication attempts.

Personal information, including that about family and friends, may also be used to fulfil another communicative function – that of *fostering social closeness*. Pages of the communication book may be devoted to introductions (for example, biographical information, a family tree and photographs) and questions to facilitate the making and maintenance of friendships. In our experience, greetings and other social forms (items that meet the requirements of *social etiquette*) are generally superfluous entries, as our clients retain other ways of communicating this information – for example, using automatic speech or natural gesture.

Having considered the type of information that may appear within a communication book, thought must obviously be given to how an individually tailored vocabulary will be devised. Wherever possible, the client should be actively involved in generating and selecting items. Those who have severe aphasia may find it useful to be offered potential categories (in an aphasia-friendly format) which they can accept or reject. Items within selected categories may then be further specified by the client's use of Total Communication (perhaps through drawing or gesturing potential entries). Other sources of inspiration may include photographs of everyday objects and events, other people's communication books and pictures from magazines. As with Total Communication, it may be useful to work with the client to draw up a weekly timetable of communication situations and partners. Vocabulary specifically aimed at these settings can then be constructed. Family and care givers may want to take part in the construction of a core vocabulary, offering ideas and helping to elucidate concepts that the person with aphasia is trying to convey.

In constructing this vocabulary, it is useful to remember that not all items have to be presented within categories, or represented by single words or phrases. Paragraph or page-length descriptions can be useful in conveying complex or highly factual information. These descriptions may include information about the client's family, personal achievements, hobbies and former employment. One of our more severely aphasic clients has created a photo-sequence within his book, detailing how he built his holiday house. Another has a page devoted to his time in the Merchant Navy.

Therapy to promote communication book use
We suggest that therapy for communication book use begins with the construction of the book and the selection of its associated vocabulary. The person with aphasia may find this process rewarding and helpful in focusing on the task ahead. If possible, the first category of items

developed should be attractive communicatively, in order to promote immediate use. Many clients choose to include items about their family initially; others may want to contribute information about a recent holiday or details of their former employment.

As soon as information appears in the book, its use should be prompted in therapy exchanges at least. The client can be asked to point to items named by the therapist to ensure all vocabulary within a designated category can be accessed. The therapist may then pose questions that can be answered by reference to the book ('Which of your daughters just got married?' 'Who did you go shopping with on Saturday?'). Structured conversations, incorporating this information, can then take place. Supported by the therapist, the client may also begin to use these details at appropriate points in group conversations. Use of the book early on, when the vocabulary is fairly small, carries the attraction of establishing interaction without the added complication of searching for items.

Early therapy should also aim to promote communication book use within the context of Total Communication, to supplement what is necessarily a limited vocabulary even when the book is relatively complete. This approach may be usefully encouraged and employed during individual and group sessions. Therapists should resist the temptation to plan sessions solely around use of the communication book, as this type of therapy has the potential to undermine development of multi-modal communication. Sessions with such a narrow remit also have a tendency to 'fall flat'. This is particularly the case in groups, where there may be insufficient common vocabulary to sustain interaction. Instead, group therapy should provide participants with opportunities to compare and discuss their books, and to develop communication strategies relevant to everyday encounters.

Working with family members and transferring skills to everyday environments

Family members may be involved in the construction of an initial vocabulary for the communication book. As the book is developed and used, family members are also likely to benefit from training to help them facilitate the aphasic person. In many respects, this training mirrors that used in generalising Total Communication and communicative drawing. PACE-type activities (Davis & Wilcox, 1985) may be used to explore and practise techniques; opportunities to observe and be observed are useful too. Specifically, those facilitating communication book users are advised to:

- Encourage use of the communication book in a variety of contexts.
- Prompt the client to always have the communication book to hand.
- Avoid extensive use of yes/no questions in conversations.
- Ask questions which require content in response.
- Allow extra time for communication.
- Prompt ('Is it in your book?') and reinforce the technique where possible.
- Encourage use of Total Communication.
- Feed back their understanding of the client's communication attempts.
- Signal when they cannot understand.
- Use situational and communicative context to interpret communication attempts (adapted from Pyatak Fletcher, 1997).

While families may provide the bridge between use of the communication book in clinical settings and its appearance in everyday communication, therapy specifically addressing this aspect may need to occur. Techniques such as those used to transfer Total Communication and communicative drawing can again be employed. One particularly useful suggestion is that a written explanation of the communication system be devised for use with others, incorporating tips for facilitation and things to avoid (Garrett *et al*, 1989; Hux *et al*, 1994).

Case Study 3.3 Using a communication book: Joe's story

At the age of 40, Joe had an extensive left-hemisphere stroke, resulting in a severe aphasia. He joined a group of people with similar impairments at the aphasia centre approximately two years ago. Prior to that, he had participated in a 12-week programme of drawing therapy. While some changes in the quality and frequency of his communicative drawing had occurred, it was obvious that his communication remained fragile. Joe had been a successful singer–songwriter. He had toured the world promoting his own work; a number of well-known recording artists regularly performed his songs. Joe's wife of eight years described him as 'eloquent' and 'fiercely Geordie'. His interests included watching Newcastle United Football Club play, and drinking the occasional pint.

Joe's auditory comprehension was relatively intact conversationally, although some deficits were noted at the single-word level during formal assessment. His spoken output was extremely limited, consisting largely of 'Aye!' and some social phrases (for example, 'Bye' and 'Thank you'). Reading comprehension was impaired at the word level. Joe was able to write his own name and some numbers. The idiosyncratic nature of his drawings meant that they could sometimes only be understood by his wife. He used a small set of spontaneous gestures to indicate guitar, keyboard, drink and cigarette. A communication aid, programmed to speak 16 short phrases, remained unused.

His involvement in the music industry effectively ceased, Joe had few interests other than watching television. He received domiciliary physiotherapy and speech and language therapy, and attended a centre for music therapy once a week. As Joe's communication skills required consolidation, and he was already making use of maps and pictographic information (including symbols from other group members' communication books) in therapy, the idea of a personalised communication book was mooted. It would provide a readily interpretable vocabulary, and could potentially be used to communicate about items that were difficult for Joe to draw (for example, song titles, favourite places). Joe expressed great interest in developing the book. He and his student keyworker agreed that they would work on it in their individual therapy sessions, and the following goal was specified:

- Joe will develop a communication book that meets his needs, in collaboration with his wife and his keyworker.

Joe's wife, however, was sceptical about the usefulness of a communication book, noting that he had been similarly keen to try his communication aid but now did not use it.

Developing the communication book

Initially, sessions were spent discussing relevant sections and potential vocabulary for the book with reference to Joe's weekly timetable, his interests and usual topics of conversation. Joe also indicated that he wanted to include all of the items from another group member's book within his own and he and the student debated the relevance of this for him. Subsequently they agreed to include sections encompassing food, drink and everyday objects (for example, sweets, Walkman). It was also decided that, in order to facilitate both Joe's and other people's access to the communication book, each vocabulary item would be represented by a drawing and a word. Joe expressed a desire to prepare all of the drawings.

A difficult period then ensued as Joe continued to express his interest in developing the book, but declined to bring any of his drawings to the sessions. This apparent reluctance continued despite a deadline for the production of the drawings being negotiated. His wife revealed that Joe did not think that his drawings were 'good enough' to appear in the book. Therapy took a new slant after she found some computer clipart and loosely arranged it in the book. This included some items that Joe had wanted to include (for example, preferred food and drink), and others that he felt were less useful.

Transferring skills to everyday environments

While his wife's actions helped to overcome one short-term problem, they were somewhat at odds with the keyworker's plan for Joe to assume primary responsibility for the development of his communication book. The student renegotiated the immediate nature of her therapy with Joe: that is, that he would indicate which items were to remain in the book, indicate how this information would be categorised and advise on the overall layout. The student's notes reveal a rekindling of Joe's interest in the book after this renegotiation. Changes included:

• Further specification of previously generic information (for example, the inclusion of the label of his favourite drink, in addition to more 'neutral' symbols for drink)

- Addition of the categories sport, events, transport, weather/seasons, days/months, therapy, and the development of corresponding vocabulary
- Inclusion of maps of the world, and of the USA
- Photographs of friends, family and favourite places
- Photographs and symbols pertaining to Newcastle United.

A key stage in the development and use of the communication book was the inclusion of information relevant to Joe's musical affairs, particularly his back catalogue, as his wife was coming under increasing pressure to release certain of his songs. She was aware that Joe held strong views about which songs should be released but, in the absence of a quick and reliable means of discussion, felt some pressure to make unilateral decisions. Small photocopies of Joe's album covers were subsequently included in the book to allow them to discuss his published work. His large catalogue of unpublished songs proved harder to accommodate; however, categorisation of these songs according to genre (for example, love song, country), and the inclusion of suitable symbols, facilitated communication. Other related information that now appears in the book includes:

- Names and photographs of fellow musicians
- Names and photographs of lyricists
- Symbols depicting certain recording labels/publishing companies
- Symbols pertaining to studio equipment
- Pictures of musical instruments

Evaluation
The following scenarios described by his wife show how, by using the communication book, Joe has regained control over aspects of his work.

1 Joe wants to tell his wife which of his tracks he wants to forward to an agent.
   Previously: Joe would gesture 'vaguely' and his wife would make a series of (often unsuccessful) guesses. Joe would find the track by listening to one of his many audio-tapes.

Now: For published work, Joe points to one of the album covers in his book, and/or a publisher's symbol and the photograph of someone he wrote it with. If the item is unpublished, Joe can point to the song's genre and/or the photograph of a collaborator.

2 Joe wants to tell his wife to phone Dave (a singer–songwriter living in California).
Previously: Joe would gesture 'phone' and point to a map of the USA. His wife would then name all of the contacts they have in the USA until she reached Dave's name.
Now: Joe gestures 'phone', and then points to Dave's photograph in the book. Before Dave's photograph was included in the book, Joe used the symbols 'man', 'singer', 'writer', as well as a map, to identify him.

Joe continues to express great interest in refining his communication book, and has recently worked on it with a new keyworker. Recent developments include information about growing up in Newcastle (using maps of the city and photographs). The student therapist has negotiated that Joe will work with his music therapist to include more technical information about recording equipment. Ultimately, Joe would like to devise some pages that function as 'stories' in their own right, which go beyond the bounds of categorised information. These include childhood memories and tales from his early days in the music industry.

Joe's wife, previously sceptical, now elaborates the book's positive contribution to everyday life. She reports that he is beginning to communicate with people who could not understand him previously, and that she is confident enough in his skills to leave him alone with others. She has noted that he can now convey complex messages, often using a combination of strategies. For example, Joe uses his communication book to specify the person he is talking about, and then drawing to 'fill in the story'.

Changes in Joe's communication, facilitated by the development and use of the communication book, have also assisted re-entry to the music business. The inclusion of album covers in his communication book has allowed him to convey decisions about the distribution of his work. He can use photographs in his book to specify which lyricists he would like to work with and, indeed, has started to collaborate musically once more. It is perhaps in his communication about musical matters that one can see another benefit of therapy emerge – that of regained identity. Joe's communication book contains many clues to his status and profession, including backstage passes, pictures of fellow musicians and album covers. He frequently uses these parts of his book when introducing himself. Joe's reference to himself as a Newcastle United supporter and Geordie further assists in asserting his identity. His wife sees the success of the communication book in these terms too: it is 'about Joe as a person'. Her occasional comment that the communication book is becoming 'Joe, This Is Your Life' may well be close to the mark.

Conversationally-based therapies

Therapies addressing communication have been transformed by advances in the theoretical understanding of conversation, and have been particularly influenced by the shift in focus from transaction to interaction. Conversation is understood to be a social act which is:

- a mundane and all-pervading form of human encounter;
- a means of establishing and maintaining relationships; and
- an interface between self and society, crucial to one's portrayal as a competent being (Levinson, 1983; Schiffrin, 1988; Wilkinson, 1995a).

A reduction in the ability to engage in conversations, as a result of aphasia, therefore has a number of disabling consequences. The person with aphasia enjoys fewer social opportunities, experiences frustration and embarrassment in conversation leading to altered relationships and reduced self-esteem (Kagan & Gailey, 1993). Within this approach, the collaborative nature of conversations is emphasised. Ongoing conversational activity is then the responsibility of all participants, as is the resolution of 'trouble spots' (Schegloff *et al*, 1977; Milroy & Perkins, 1992; Goodwin, 1995).

Correspondingly, there has been a broadening of therapies at the conversational level, from those focusing on aspects of the aphasic person's ability – for example, turn taking and repair (Davis & Wilcox, 1985; Pulvermuller & Roth, 1991; Leiwo, 1994) – to others addressing the skills of non-aphasic interactants and the communication partnership as a whole (for example, Lesser & Algar, 1995; Wilkinson, 1995b; Wilkinson *et al*, 1998; Booth & Perkins, 1999; Booth & Swabey, 1999). A focus on conversation as a medium for social involvement has also lead to concerted efforts to create supportive conversational environments for aphasic people; Aura Kagan and Jon Lyon are pioneers in this field. Their work, addressing Supported Conversation and the involvement of Communication Partners respectively, is rapidly becoming established as part of the therapeutic approach to aphasia.

Supported Conversation and
working with communication partners

Drawing on insights provided by certain conversation analysts (for example, Schiffrin, 1988), the therapeutic approach known as Supported Conversation for Adults with Aphasia (SCA) (Kagan & Gailey, 1993; Kagan, 1998) is underpinned by the idea that competence can be revealed by conversation itself. According to this view, ongoing conversational activity is crucial to one's being perceived as capable by others. Aphasia, with its capacity to disrupt conversational fluency, may serve to 'mask' an individual's competence. As a result, the aphasic person's ability to make decisions may be called into question, as may his or her ability to participate in everyday discussions. The person with impaired language may be excluded from a variety of communicative situations by non-aphasic communication partners. Kagan (1995) argues that such a restriction in 'communicative access' has implications for the psychological health and well-being of aphasic individuals.

Supported Conversation attempts to redress these consequences, and reveal the inherent competence of aphasic people, by creating appropriately facilitative environments. This includes the training of non-aphasic people in Supported Conversation techniques (as shown in Table

3.3) and the use of aphasia-friendly material to augment verbal communication – for example, the *Pictographic Communication Resources Manual* (Kagan *et al*, 1996). The provision of space and time for aphasic people to converse is important within this approach; again, Kagan's volunteer-led conversation groups for aphasic people have been described elsewhere (for example, Kagan & Gailey, 1993).

Table 3.3 *Supported Conversation techniques*

To facilitate comprehension, the clinician may ...	*To facilitate output, the clinician may ...*
Use pictures, objects, and/or written words to supplement speech	Encourage Total Communication and accept any modality offered
Use natural gesture and drawing in communication	Provide relevant pictures, objects and/or written information for client use
Modify aspects of his or her speech, eg, by slowing rate, emphasising key words	Allow extra time for responses
Allow extra time for the processing of information	Use Total Communication strategies themselves
Signal speaker change by using gaze or natural gesture	Facilitate sharing of the 'floor' (eg, by passing turns to less active participants)
Signal topic change through the use of Total Communication	Encourage client–client interactions by verbally linking group members
Verbally confirm (clients') unclear messages for group members	Facilitate topic change when the topic at hand is flagging

Source: adapted from Kagan & Gailey (1993)

In addition, steps are taken to create the 'feel and flow' of natural conversation. These include using humour conversationally; periodically verifying the aphasic person's message; and verbally linking members during group interactions. By training others to use these 'communication ramps', Kagan hopes to improve aphasic individuals' access to everyday interactions, and their participation in satisfying conversations in which their competence is both revealed and acknowledged.

In working with Communication Partners, Lyon *et al* (1997) also acknowledge the importance of conversation within everyday life, particularly in the maintenance of well-being and self-esteem. This approach also involves the training of non-aphasic volunteers in communication techniques. It is different to SCA, however, in that it involves a one-to-one pairing of volunteer and aphasic person rather than group encounters. This one-to-one pairing provides several advantages, including the development of personally relevant communication strategies, continuity of contact and befriending.

A key feature of this therapy is the use of conversation, and the communication partnership, as a vehicle for reintegration: once effective communication has been established, the communication partner is encouraged to collaborate with the aphasic partner to identify opportunities for participation in the local community. These opportunities may include activities that the person enjoyed before the onset of aphasia, and no longer pursues, or new ventures (for example, playing tennis or going to the cinema). The Communication Partner becomes a facilitator, assisting the aphasic person physically, communicatively and/or organisationally to engage in these activities.

Lyon *et al* (1997) see the benefits of such an approach in the creation of real-life communication opportunities, if not during the selected activity, then later as the aphasic person relates new experiences to friends and family. Communicative confidence may increase through repeated encounters with a skilled and supportive conversation partner. Importantly, the aphasic person's sense of self may be enhanced as the focus falls upon involvement and ability rather than disability. This approach has the potential to 'alter [an aphasic individual's] view of himself and what [is] possible in life' (Lyon *et al*, 1997, p695).

Conversationally-based therapies at the aphasia centre

Therapy at the conversational level takes a number of forms at the centre. It may follow a traditional approach, by addressing the aphasic person's ability to take turns and contribute to repair (*see* Table 3.4 for some sample aims and methods), or by facilitating the transfer of new communication skills (for example, communicative drawing) to everyday interactions. Therapy may also address the actions of habitual conversation partnerships. Our interventions involving people with aphasia and their families often incorporate elements of 'interaction therapy' in which the therapist guides partnerships through videotapes of their conversations, and facilitates discussion of potential and achievable modifications to their interactions (Wilkinson, 1995b; Wilkinson *et al*, 1998). Parallel techniques such as PACE (Davis & Wilcox, 1985) and Conversational Coaching may then be employed to effect change.

Our own conversationally-based therapies also branch out from the approaches described above. While highly influenced by the work of Kagan and Lyon, the Conversation Group and Conversation Partners programme have been tailored to the needs of our clients and according to our resources. For example, the Conversation Group is primarily comprised of people with mild to moderate aphasia. It is also facilitated by student speech and language therapists and (more recently) aphasic group members, instead of volunteers. Similarly, the non-aphasic participants in the Conversation Partners scheme are recruited from our student body rather than the local community.

The Conversation Group

The Conversation Group at the aphasia centre was developed with the aim of providing aphasic people with an environment in which to engage in satisfying conversations. A core group of eight members meet for one and a half hours per week to engage in themed conversations. Group members generally have mild to moderate aphasia, although two individuals have severely restricted verbal output. Despite some group members' relatively preserved language, all report difficulty conversing in everyday contexts, coupled with anxiety and embarrassment. As well as opportunities to participate in supported conversations, the group

Table 3.4 *Methods in therapy for turntaking*

Therapy aims	Example methods
1 Group members will agree component behaviours of effective turn taking	• Group members watch videos and therapist-led role plays of 'good' and 'bad' conversations, identifying behaviours that influence turn taking (comedy programmes can be a particularly useful source of 'bad' turn taking) • Group members consider their everyday conversations, identifying behaviours that influence turn taking. The videos/role plays may be used as a point of reference (that is, 'does X happen to you?'). Group members also discuss the feelings they experience when unable to get a turn • The group agrees a core set of effective turn taking behaviours and standard icons to represent these. (This group chose to focus on *eye contact*; *listening*; *one person at a time* [that is, avoiding competing turns]; and *staying on topic*)
2 Group members will monitor the use of these behaviours in others' conversations	• Group members watch videos of others' conversations ('good' and 'bad'). They use a checklist to identify which of the turn taking behaviours were present/absent • Group members watch therapist-led role plays of 'bad' turn taking. They use a diagram of the standard icons to indicate which aspects were in 'error' and suggest areas for change. These changes are incorporated within a re-run of the role play

continued

Table 3.4 *continued*

3 Group members will apply and monitor the use of these behaviours in their own conversations	• The group has a short conversation on a selected topic. Prior to the conversation, each group member identifies a turn taking behaviour that he or she wishes to use and monitor. Afterwards, each person rates personal use of the behaviour • As for above task, but the other group members are asked to comment on (a) whether the behaviour was present and (b) how effectively it was used. Videorecording the conversation may assist the monitoring process
4 Group members will each identify and practise two strategies that assist in 'getting into' conversations	• Group members brainstorm different ways of getting into conversations. Again, video and role play may be used to illustrate a range of options • Each group member selects one strategy that they would like to try in a role play (this may be one that they already use, or something new). They rate the effectiveness of this strategy. A second strategy is then trialled in this way • The method above can also be used conversationally. The therapist may use Conversational Coaching with the group as a whole (eg, stopping the conversation at certain points to discuss proceedings/suggest areas for change) or with certain individuals

provides a forum for members to discuss the effect of aphasia upon everyday interactions. Group members are keen to use their experience to inform others; for example, they are currently compiling a leaflet addressing stroke, aphasia and conversations to educate family, friends and strangers.

Background information
Formed just over two years ago, the Conversation Group followed on from a well-received therapy programme addressing conversation skills, and was underpinned by group members' keenness to engage in conversations in a supportive setting. It was also motivated by the writings of Kagan and Gailey (1993). Facilitated by a speech and language therapist, and comprising several members from our therapy groups, the Conversation Group was initially limited in its success. This was due, in part, to sporadic attendance: clients who attended therapy groups two days a week were sometimes unable to come in for another morning. Group members also appeared to have difficulty divorcing this new venture from other groups. While they were encouraged to interact with each other, and were verbally linked by the SLT during conversations, much of their communication was directed to the therapist. One group member repeatedly expressed a desire to work on his writing during the group's meetings. This Conversation Group was, sadly, disbanded after two months.

After a period of reflection, the group was re-formed approximately three months later. In light of the difficulty the original members had in differentiating the Conversation Group from mainstream therapy groups, it was decided that only those who had left therapy would be invited to join. Consequently, the six members of our self-help group were asked to form the core of the new Conversation Group. In order to facilitate these members' attendance, the new group was scheduled on the same day as their meetings. Three other people, who were not involved in the self-help or original conversation group, were also invited to join at this time.

As the self-help group was already well established, it was hoped that their patterns of interaction would ensure that conversations would take place with less reference to the therapist. In fact, it was envisioned that, after an initial period of facilitation, members would take on aspects of the group's organisation (for example, identifying topics for themed conversations, gathering related materials) and ultimately assume responsibility for running the Conversation Group. We were aware that this approach would pose certain challenges to group members, but felt that it would distinguish the Conversation Group from other groups run at the centre, promote more naturalistic exchanges and foster mutual support.

Becoming an established group

As soon as the new Conversation Group started meeting, it was clear they had the potential to function more independently than the first group. Existing patterns of interaction meant that the group did converse with less reference to the therapist present. Self-help group members were already undertaking certain organisational tasks (for example, collecting subscription money, organising outings) in the running of their group. It was apparent, however, that the group was having difficulty accommodating the communication skills of two new members with more severe aphasia – one of whom had markedly impaired auditory comprehension. These two group members, and another severely aphasic person already attending the self-help group, were often excluded from conversations unless the therapist intervened. Other interactional difficulties arose as two fluent group members tended to take very long turns. Several group members (new and old) expressed their dissatisfaction with this.

While the therapist was keen not to assume a central role in the group's meetings, it was obvious that, unless these difficulties were dealt with directly, the Conversation Group was in danger of losing some participants. With the agreement of the group, she subsequently coordinated several sessions in which they were facilitated to consider the nature of conversation, the basics of turn taking, and helpful and unhelpful conversational behaviours. During these sessions, group members discussed (for example) the need to have pens and paper to hand in all sessions, in order to facilitate those members who used writing and/or drawing in their communication. The need to use gesture and writing, where possible, to assist members with auditory comprehension problems was also broached. It was during these sessions that the idea that group members could play a role in the education of non-aphasic people was first mooted.

While it was apparent that some group members benefited from these sessions, in that their interactions with others were generally more facilitatory (for example, offering pen and paper where necessary), some members continued with less helpful interaction strategies. Long turns were, again, particularly disruptive. In addition, while the therapist expressed the wish that group members would ultimately organise and run the group, few felt able to do so at this stage. The group members and the therapist agreed that some speech and language therapy input (for example, assistance in facilitating less able members, help in dealing with group dynamics) would continue in the short term. As the therapist's ability to take a 'back seat' in group meeting had been undermined by the need to resolve some communication issues, it was decided that she would no longer regularly attend the group. Rather, speech and language therapy students would be recruited to provide the group with practical assistance.

Current issues for the Conversation Group

Since this time, the group has met regularly during university terms. Five of the original nine group members continue to attend most sessions. As planned, student speech and language therapists have often assisted in the group's organisation. At present, the group is dividing its time between having conversations and preparing the leaflet. Not all has gone smoothly, however: group members are still some way from running the group autonomously and interactional problems continue to arise. At present, as at certain points in the past, the group is grappling with issues related to group composition and function. In particular, tensions are created by the presence of therapists in the group; some reluctance on the part of aphasic group members to become more actively involved; and the broad range of communication skills represented.

Involvement of therapists in the group

The involvement of student therapists, while conferring a number of benefits, has also posed some problems for group function. This is due in part to some group members being unable to understand the supportive, rather than actively therapeutic, role that the students have assumed. They comment: 'You decide, you're the boss'. Student therapists have also had difficulty in delineating their involvement. In order to define her role within the group, one student identified the following goals for participation:

Student therapists will facilitate group members in achieving natural conversation by:

- Providing necessary 'props' to conversation (for example, pens, paper, pictures)
- Having a knowledge of conversational conventions and using these to promote interaction (for example, assisting in flagging up topic changes, dealing with competing turns)
- Having a knowledge of how aphasia affects conversation and how to manage its effects (for example, by promoting Total Communication, involving less active/able members)
- Encouraging group members to select and debate topics
- Being client-led (for example, in terms of topics selected and pursued).

Adherence to these guidelines has helped to enhance the contributions of group members, and create an appropriately facilitative environment. Aphasic participants now have more access to the conversational floor. Corresponding efforts by student therapists to reduce their involvement in the topic at hand and focus more on the supportive aspects of their role have also lead to an increase in client–client (instead of client–therapist) interactions.

Involvement of aphasic group members
Linked with efforts to define therapist involvement in the group, and a move away from therapist-mediated intervention, continued attempts have been made to increase members' participation in all aspects of the Conversation Group. While most remain reluctant to assist in running the group, two group members have recently volunteered their help in

planning and executing sessions. Earlier efforts to involve these and other members in the group's organisation included the following guidelines:

1   Group members are encouraged to decide, at the end of each session, the agenda for the following week – for example, whether to have conversations, work on the leaflet or do both. If a conversation is selected, group members are facilitated to consider potential topics and whether to have this conversation in small or large groups.
2   Student therapists consult with the two aphasic co-facilitators at the end of each session regarding the success or otherwise of that session. Members are asked to feed back on those aspects that went well, and those that could have been improved. Other issues arising from the session (for example, problems including less verbal members) are also discussed. The co-facilitators are encouraged to suggest ways of dealing with these. The students then incorporate their aphasic partners' suggestions within plans for subsequent sessions.
3   One of the aphasic group members takes and/or types up minutes generated within the session (for example, decisions about the content and layout of the leaflet). This person assumes responsibility for ensuring that these minutes are distributed to other group members.

The involvement of the two aphasic co-facilitators seems to have had a positive effect upon aspects of group functioning. One co-facilitator has demonstrated an ability to include less able or active members of the group conversationally, by seeking their opinions and/or offering pen and paper to encourage drawn or written communication. Both are becoming more assertive in their requests for the group to keep on topic, particularly when the leaflet is being discussed.

This increased involvement by members is now allowing therapy staff to reduce their input to the group; again, within-group interactions have increased accordingly. Student therapists still lend practical support, as required. The nature of this support is negotiated during feedback sessions with the aphasic co-facilitators, and may include the preparation of materials for themed conversations, help in facilitating a group member's communication, or assistance in finding suitable accommodation for the group. A recent request has been for the students to develop an aphasia-friendly timetable, so that the co-facilitators can explain the timing and sequencing of meetings to other group members.

Communication skills

As already explained, while most group members have mild to moderate aphasia, some have more severely impaired language. Although there are some facilitatory techniques that may be useful for both sets of clients, there are others that are specific to each group. For example, clients who are fluent may need facilitation to curtail inappropriately long turns. Clients with more marked difficulties may need support to use alternative or augmentative methods in their interactions. While aphasia therapists should be flexible enough to facilitate people with different levels of impairment, differences in the speed and efficiency of these clients' communication may make mixed-ability groups problematic. These difficulties may be compounded if, as in the case of the Conversation Group, the group facilitators have aphasia themselves. The nature of the facilitators' aphasia may mean (say) that they are unable to write messages to a group member with impaired auditory but spared reading comprehension.

Interactional problems do arise in the group as a result of some mismatch in group members' communication skills. Without careful facilitation, there is a tendency for more able members to dominate conversations, with the corresponding exclusion of clients with more fragile skills. One group member who has markedly impaired auditory comprehension reports that he sometimes is frustrated by his inability to follow the talk of other members. The additional time that more severely impaired communicators take to make their contributions may also serve to frustrate others. Loss of the conversational floor may occur as a more able group member assumes the turn. As the Conversation Group gains more members, it may be useful to create a separate group for people with severe aphasia, so that they can be given extra time and facilitation in the pursuit of rewarding conversations. Having said this, the obvious engagement and enjoyment experienced by some of our severely aphasic clients when in mixed-ability groups means that decisions regarding involvement should probably be made on an individual basis, and with reference to current group needs and dynamics.

Evaluation

Despite these difficulties, many members enjoy being part of the group. This enjoyment may stem from regular contact with friends. Group members also find themed conversations intellectually stimulating, as the following comments show:

> 'Yes, it's quite excitable, isn't it ... somebody gets quite ... some – something that's happened – that's being discussed by everyone ... you know we've had some quite ... *interesting* subjects, haven't we? ... um ... yes, one gets genuinely quite excited ... you know what I mean ... whatever it's about.'

> 'Any ... um ... speaking out all the time ... no ... maybe the ... no cobwebs ... in the brain.'

Group members also comment that conversations within the group are more pleasurable, and less anxiety-provoking, than interactions in the outside world. Some group members report changes in their confidence since joining:

> 'Better ... maybe ... I think, I dunno ... long time ago ... first stroke, as in ... [forearm held to chest, fist clenched] ... shy all the time ... and drawn ... but maybe 'spress [head flung back, large circular movement with arm to whole group] in conversation ... all the time ... is much better.'

Others value the opportunity for their competence to be revealed in a supportive environment:

> 'I think it's great actually, actually ... you're the sort of per-person that you remember what sort of person we are ... you remember what we are, and you don't forget that ... it's important sometimes ... some people, they don't remember *me*.'

Group members also enjoy their role as expert conversationalists. Several group projects, all with an educational slant, have been

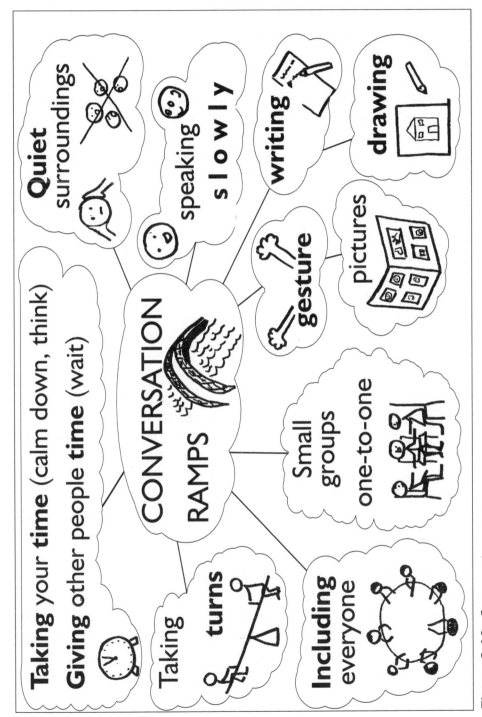

Figure 3.10 *Conversation ramps*

suggested as a follow-on to the leaflet. These include an introductory pack explaining aphasia and its effects on conversations for first-year speech and language therapy students. The group is also keen to develop a resource file (containing pictographic and other material) to facilitate the conversations of other people with aphasia. Figure 3.10, for example, illustrates the range of conversation ramps that group members may use when engaging in conversations. These suggestions have been warmly received and it is anticipated that materials produced by the group will be routinely used within the centre. When considering such project work, it is apparent that the Conversation Group is beginning to confer benefits beyond opportunities for pleasurable interactions. In providing an environment in which to be creative and business-like, and in which contributions are valued, the group may promote engagement and involvement within the community of the aphasia centre.

Conversation Partners

Our Conversation Partners scheme has also been running for about two years and takes its lead from the programme conceived by Lyon and colleagues (Lyon et al, 1997). The scheme was developed in conjunction with speech and language therapists employed by Camden and Islington Community Health Services NHS Trust in London. It is specifically designed to meet the needs of people with long-term aphasia who are socially disadvantaged by a lack of skilled conversation partners. Conversation Partners aims to reduce the social isolation that may accompany aphasia. This change may initially be effected through contact, at home, between the person with aphasia and a trained volunteer. As the partnership develops and the partners venture further afield, involvement in community groups and local recreational activities may help to bring about social re-engagement.

Our scheme differs from that described by Lyon et al (1997) in that we use student speech and language therapists as volunteer conversation partners. This is not to say that volunteers from the local community are not involved in the scheme. When available, they can prove invaluable because of their first-hand knowledge of the area, and corresponding ability to access a range of community services. We have found, however, that such volunteers are often in short supply.

It has also been our experience that student therapists, while perhaps lacking local knowledge, more than make up for this in terms of enthusiasm. To date, we have largely focused on involving first-year undergraduates in the programme, as at this stage of their studies they have relatively light clinical commitments. Student speech and language therapists also have the advantage over community volunteers that they are interested in working with people with communication impairments. In addition, they are already receiving theoretical and practical support in understanding the principles and practice of human communication. All volunteer Conversation Partners are asked to commit two hours per fortnight to the scheme for at least six months.

The training that we provide our Conversation Partners aims to consolidate their knowledge of communication, and enable them to interact effectively with people who have aphasia. Each volunteer attends two group training sessions before meeting his or her aphasic partner. In these sessions, aphasia is described, its communicative and social consequences outlined, and basic communication techniques are introduced. The sessions also elaborate the anticipated benefits of the Conversation Partners scheme. Time is spent teasing out differences between this scheme and more traditional speech and language therapy. Volunteers are strongly advised that their remit is to be a conversation partner and not a therapist.

Each volunteer's first encounter with his or her aphasic partner is then videotaped. The encounter is subsequently reviewed in a meeting between the volunteer and a speech and language therapist attached to the scheme, in order to further specify relevant communication strategies. In addition to these initial training sessions, the Conversation Partners meet monthly, as a group and with therapy staff, to share experiences and brainstorm solutions to problems. These sessions may also address ways of accessing local resources. Contact between volunteers and therapists, in the form of regular supervision meetings and telephone calls, is also maintained throughout the scheme.

To date, our experience with the Conversation Partners scheme has been largely positive. Ten conversation partnerships have been created. Aphasic participants have included those living in their own homes and others living in residential-care settings (for example, warden-controlled accommodation and nursing homes). Most of these people have severe aphasia; one participant has mildly impaired language. While conversations at home form the basis of most encounters, some partnerships have ventured out into the community. Feedback from aphasic participants and volunteers has been encouraging. People with aphasia indicate that they enjoy and anticipate the Conversation Partner's visits, while volunteers report a greater understanding of aphasia and its outcomes, and a deeper respect for aphasic people.

Family members have expressed their appreciation for the social contact that the scheme affords their aphasic relative. One participant's daughter noted that her mother seemed happier and more relaxed during the volunteer's visits. Perhaps understandably, our students have at times come under pressure to provide a speech and language therapy service. They have required continued support to explain their role and establish their presence as Conversation Partners.

Case Study 3.4 Conversation Partners: George and Sophie's story

George is a retired sailor aged 66 years. He had a stroke five years ago, which resulted in aphasia. George's communication is severely restricted. Some problems with auditory comprehension are apparent conversationally, and his spoken output primarily consists of 'yes', 'no' and certain expletives. His reading and writing are impaired at the single-word level. George is unable to draw communicatively and his gestures tend to be non-specific. He is able to vocalise, however, and can use intonation to express emotions and preferences. He also employs facial expression and pointing during communication attempts. George has a hemiplegia and uses a wheelchair.

George lives at home with his wife, Rose. He spends much of his day watching television, and has no visitors beyond his immediate family. Until a recent bout of ill health, his only regular social contact came through a local Stroke Club, which he attended once a week.

George was introduced to his Conversation Partner, Sophie, approximately 16 months ago. Sophie is 24 years old, comes from

Greece and is studying Speech and Language Therapy at City University. She is a naturally warm and engaging communicator, although her first videotaped conversation with George revealed a tendency to take long turns and speak too quickly. She also assumed most of the responsibility for initiating interaction, was keen to fill silences, and did not always notice George's communication attempts. While Sophie had brought along some photographs to facilitate the conversation, they reflected her own interests and were consequently of limited relevance to George. Upon reviewing the video, Sophie and her supervising clinician agreed that she would:

- Slow her rate of speech
- Take shorter turns
- Allow silences within conversation
- Let George 'take the lead' conversationally – for example, allowing him to initiate topics
- Use visual material that reflected George's interests

Sophie was also concerned that Rose tended to monopolise her time with George. She decided that, in the first instance, she would make a concerted effort to direct her communication to George. If this difficulty continued, she planned to reiterate the purpose of her visits.

As anticipated, these methods provided George with more opportunities to contribute to conversations. In particular, Sophie's use of relevant visual material proved successful. For example, George used the maps she brought to show the countries he had been to while in the Navy, and to plot specific voyages. Picture books about the countryside also sparked conversations, with George pointing to pleasant scenes and places that he had visited. He also enjoyed looking at books on architecture, and indicated that Sophie should bring some information about Greece. Sophie's increased tolerance of silences also allowed George to initiate and add content to exchanges, resulting in a greater sharing of conversational turns. She remarked that conversations consequently became more interesting. As George became more able to participate, and Sophie directed much communication towards him, Rose began to busy herself elsewhere during visits.

Over the course of time, George and Sophie's sessions began, naturally, to follow two main themes. The first part of each visit was devoted to discussing the previous week's news, while the second part involved looking at maps and books. They would sometimes watch George's favourite television programme, a cookery challenge in which well-known chefs prepare a range of dishes in a short period of time. Conversations during and after the programme would focus on the meals produced, with George indicating the dishes he liked and why they appealed to him. During their sessions, George and Sophie also discovered a mutual passion for a particular type of sweet available only at Woolworth's. Weather permitting, they began to make regular forays to the local store. Sophie reported that George looked forward to these trips.

George's anticipation of these trips was, according to his wife, matched by his enthusiasm for Sophie's visits. She indicated that he had become noticeably happier since Sophie had begun to call. George's wife also reported that he looked through the books that Sophie left between visits, and used the maps to reminisce about his time as a sailor. He became interested in doing jigsaw puzzles, especially those depicting country scenes. George's renewed interest in his past lead to he, his wife and Sophie compiling a time line of his life. This time line included information about when and where George and Rose were married, when their children were born, and when he joined the Navy. Sophie also noticed some changes in George over the course of their contact. In particular, she felt that he assumed the role of protector, concerned for her welfare, and keen to warn of the dangers associated with living in London.

Unfortunately, George and Sophie's sessions have stopped for the time being due to his ill health. Sophie feels strongly that she has benefited from her time with George. Apart from the communication skills that she has acquired, Sophie reports a heightened awareness of the everyday effects of aphasia. She also states that she has a greater appreciation of the life experience and world knowledge that people with aphasia bring to interactions. In Sophie's opinion, she has benefited from her contact with George's wife too. A continued challenge has been to explain her role as a Conversation Partner rather than a speech and language therapist. George's wife has recently asked Sophie to carry out a number of therapy-like tasks, including speech and reading exercises. This is an issue that will need to be addressed when George and Sophie resume contact. A further challenge will arise in a few months' time, when Sophie qualifies as a therapist and returns to Greece. We hope to find a similarly skilled and warm volunteer in order to perpetuate a mutually beneficial partnership.

CHAPTER 4

Breaking Down the Barriers

External and internal barriers

In Chapter 1, we outlined a relatively new conceptual framework that has profoundly influenced our understanding of and approach to aphasia therapy: the social model of disability. This model represents disability in terms of the socially constructed barriers which spring up around people with impairments, rather than as directly resulting from the impairment itself. Examples of some of the external barriers which people with aphasia face were described, and these can be categorised in terms of environmental, structural, attitudinal and informational factors. In keeping with this conceptualisation of aphasia, we try to work together with clients to address the socially constructed limitations of opportunity which they face. This accords with the proposal by French (1994, p15) that professionals should 'act as supportive enablers, actively sharing their expertise and knowledge while recognising the expertise of disabled people and learning from them.'

According to proponents of the social model, professionals concerned with disability face an imperative to shift their focus away from helping 'disabled people to cope and adapt in a society adapted to the needs of non-disabled people' (French, 1993, p45), and instead work with disabled people towards identifying and removing the barriers which exist. This conceptual shift is perhaps most readily understood in terms of the experience of people with mobility impairments. If the environment could be made physically accessible through the improved design of buildings, more accessible transport systems and free availability of whatever mobility aid or personal assistance an individual requires, then that person's mobility problems would effectively cease to exist. Disability is socially created and imposed, not inherent.

Following this argument to its full conclusion leads to the suggestion that therapists should cease attempting to effect change in the individual's impairment and focus instead upon changing the environment. This argument has been considered in the context of language impairment.

> [If] disability is defined entirely in terms of barriers ... removing such barriers is seen as an essential prerequisite for the empowerment of aphasic people. (Jordan & Kaiser, 1996, p139)

Thus, many of the disabling consequences of aphasia might be removed if service providers and the general public ceased to hold attitudes which stigmatise those with communication impairments. If service providers were trained to facilitate communication, if advocates were easily accessible to aphasic people, if information could be routinely provided in a range of aphasia-friendly formats, if background noise were kept to a minimum in all places where aphasic people might need to communicate, the disability associated with aphasia would be greatly reduced.

However, such changes are slow to effect, depend on mass collective action and are unlikely ever to be fully achieved. People with aphasia must still operate within environments and systems which are less than ideal. In addition, it is important to acknowledge that many disabled people understand their impairments in terms of the culturally dominant medical model of disability. This may be particularly true in the case of people with aphasia, since 'theories and campaigns relating to disability have been largely inaccessible to people who have language impairment' (Parr et al, 1997, p133). The internalisation of medical model constructs may decrease a person's confidence and self-esteem, and lead to a sense of powerlessness. These constitute internal barriers to autonomy. Therapists face the challenge of addressing barriers at a societal level while at the same time supporting individual clients in coping with the internal and external barriers that do exist. There is no straightforward solution to this complex issue, but it seems that a flexible approach, in which clients and those around them are assisted to develop effective communication (as described in Chapter 3) while also addressing socially constructed barriers, provides the best way forward.

Addressing barriers: approaches to therapy

Taken in a literal sense, a barrier constitutes a physical obstruction which impedes a person's opportunity to reach a desired situation or goal. By analogy, therapy that addresses barriers in order to enable that person to achieve the desired situation or goal can take one of three approaches. Therapist and client work together in order to:

- climb over the barrier
- find a way round the barrier
- dismantle and remove the barrier

Climbing over the barrier is analogous to developing the individual's own skills and abilities – for example, by improving language skills through psycholinguistically motivated therapies, or by developing communication and conversational skills. In other words, it adheres to traditional models of impairment-based therapy. *Finding a way around the barrier* might, for instance, involve work on the development of strategies and the use of aids such as the personalised communication books, as described in Chapter 3, or the use of technology to bypass some aspects of the individual's language processing impairment.

Work on *dismantling and removing barriers* is less straightforward, and can operate at micro and macro levels. For instance, the communication style of a family member or friend may constitute a barrier to the aphasic person's participation in conversation. This barrier might be dismantled, at least partially, through specific therapy that assists the non-aphasic person to adopt a more facilitative communication style. Other forms of barrier, such as those created by culturally dominant negative attitudes towards disability, or by organisational structures and policies, will only be addressed adequately through sustained collective action in the form of campaigning, political lobbying, education and awareness raising. Inevitably, this depends on the development of a collective identity among people with aphasia – an issue which is addressed in Chapter 5.

In reality, much of the therapy that we offer integrates all these approaches. Thus, therapy primarily aimed at improving an individual's communication skills is likely to have implications also for their confidence and self-esteem as well as better equipping them to deal with the barriers to communication and participation which they face. Equally, therapy aimed primarily at increasing a person's assertiveness will bring about changes to their communication skills, and may well result indirectly in a reduction in the barriers created by the patronising attitudes of others towards them. In this chapter, we outline a range of therapies that focus primarily on the disabling external and internal barriers encountered by people with aphasia, but which inevitably draw on and contribute to changes in our clients' communication skills and personal identity.

Overcoming external barriers: project therapy

In recent years, clients attending the centre have become increasingly involved in project therapy. Project therapy is particularly suitable for groupwork, but it can also be useful and beneficial to clients working on an individual basis. Recent projects include:

- Making videos to teach primary school children and speech and language therapy students respectively about the nature and consequences of aphasia
- Organising group outings to museums, restaurants and places of interest
- Producing an aphasia-friendly leaflet, map and travel directions to the centre for new group members
- Writing an aphasia-friendly recipe book designed for one-handed cooks

Projects can take many forms and be implemented in different ways, but share some common features:

- Clients determine the project aims
- Clients take control at all stages of decision making
- During project sessions the therapist acts primarily as a facilitator and advocate
- Projects provide opportunities for clients to practise communication skills and strategies both within and outside the clinical setting

It is widely acknowledged that communication therapy should aim for generalisation of skills developed within the clinic to the 'real world' (for example, Kagan & Gailey, 1993; Green, 1984), although this is not always straightforward or easily achieved. Problems in establishing real-life communication skills and strategies may be due in part to the contrived nature of many interactions set up in therapy sessions, and to the difference in contextual constraints that exist between clinical and 'real world' situations (Oxenham, 1994). A client may find that skills and strategies that are ably and confidently used in a quiet therapy room with a facilitative therapist prove elusive when faced with the demands of communicating with a stranger in a noisy environment and in front of several curious onlookers (*see* Chapter 3 for a more detailed discussion of these issues). Project-based therapy addresses some of the problems of carry-over by creating opportunities for clients to use their skills in non-contrived situations (though still with the appropriate level of support). It can bridge the gap between the clinic and the real world.

Project work has several other advantages which distinguish it from traditional functional therapy. These relate to a number of issues concerning the client's autonomy and engagement.

1 *Autonomy*

Project therapy provides an effective means of promoting clients' autonomy and developing an ethos of self-help. Unlike traditional therapy, in which the therapist ordinarily sets the agenda and controls what happens, in project work the client takes responsibility for all project-related decisions. The therapist has limited say over what the project will be or how it will be carried out (except in the unlikely event that there is significant risk of harm to the client). This feature of project work can be particularly important in enabling clients to release themselves from the 'sick role', and to begin to counter the damaging loss of control which can occur with the onset of aphasia (Jordan & Kaiser, 1996). Taking responsibility for decision making encourages clients to employ a problem-solving approach which they can generalise to other real-life situations. By handing over control of the project, the therapist explicitly acknowledges the competence of the person with aphasia.

2   *Engagement in therapy*
People who attend the centre seem to be highly motivated and engaged by working on projects. Clients set project goals that they find interesting and meaningful, and this creates a real desire for the project to be carried out. Project work also calls up a genuine need for communication, far beyond that which exists in artificial communication tasks. The powerful, motivating force of a project is often manifested in the dynamic, client-initiated interactions which can take place in project sessions (and which can sometimes be lacking in therapist-initiated discussions). Clients willingly set themselves challenging assignments (such as making a telephone call to obtain information that is needed for a project decision) that they might have avoided taking on had there been no real need for the task to be carried out.

3   *Group dynamic*
Project work can quickly lead to a positive group dynamic being established as group members appreciate that their common goals can only be achieved through cooperation and mutual support. This positive ethos often carries over into other non-project therapy sessions.

4   *The rewarding nature of project work*
Project work usually has a real and tangible outcome or product (for example, a leaflet, a video or an outing) which can be highly affirming and reinforcing. The successful culmination of a project that has been worked on collaboratively for a number of weeks or months provides a natural point at which to take stock of progress and an opportunity for clients to acknowledge what they have achieved.

Distinguishing therapeutic and project aims

There is a distinction to be made between the practical and therapeutic levels on which a project operates. Therapeutic aims relate to the personal or functional changes that clients are intending to make as a result of the project therapy, but are not confined to any specific project. These may be shared by the whole group or specific to individuals. The same therapeutic aims can be achieved by very different kinds of project, but of course clients need to be clear about their aims and the kinds of opportunity that they require when they are choosing a project.

Thus, if one *therapeutic aim* concerns building confidence in requesting information from strangers, only limited opportunities to achieve this might be created by a primarily clinic-based project such as writing a leaflet. However, a project in which group members organise a trip to a restaurant could provide numerous opportunities for communication with strangers. *Project aims* are more specific and practical and act as the vehicle for therapeutic aims. Thus, for a visit to a restaurant, project aims might include finding out about wheelchair access, menus, prices and transport facilities from a number of establishments. This in turn would create opportunities to practise strategies for requesting information from strangers (either in person or by telephone), thus enabling clients to work towards the therapeutic aim of building confidence in this area.

The role of the therapist in project work

The role of the therapist in project work is subtly different to that in traditional therapy. Rather than taking responsibility for planning, organising and directing activity, the therapist acts primarily as a facilitator for the clients. This may involve:

- Assisting clients in identifying realistic and appropriate therapeutic aims, and providing feedback in relation to those aims during project sessions
- Facilitating clients' communication during discussions and assisting in repair of conversational breakdown
- Helping clients to problem-solve, and to identify and practise useful communication strategies

- Recording information about the project, often in the form of aphasia-friendly minutes of meetings (as in Chapter 1, Figure 1.2)
- Acting as an advocate, where necessary, for the attainment of project goals – for instance, by writing a formal letter under the explicit direction of the group members

---

Case Study 4.1 The stroke and aphasia leaflet project

Clients with severe language impairments worked together on a project producing personalised leaflets designed to raise awareness of stroke and aphasia. On numerous occasions prior to the group project it had been apparent that the group members did not have a clear understanding of the nature of stroke and aphasia, due perhaps to the paucity of information available in accessible formats. It was clear that they wished to know more about what had happened to them. It was also apparent that group members had limited means of explaining their impairments and needs to people they met outside the centre. The group therefore decided to spend a weekly session over the course of one term exploring the nature and effects of stroke and aphasia. Group members also wanted to gather resources that would assist them in raising awareness of stroke and aphasia.

For group members, the therapeutic aims were:

1 To adapt to changed communication
2 To make more use of alternative means of communication
3 To raise levels of self-confidence
4 To effect changes in the environments in which they needed to communicate

In order for group members and those around them to change, they had to access relevant information, in this case regarding stroke illness and aphasia. Group sessions involved members sharing information and ideas through brainstorming and facilitated discussion to establish what they already understood and to enable them to share their personal experiences of stroke and aphasia. Student key workers also provided accurate information in accessible formats – for example, noting down facts on the whiteboard in key words, pictograms and familiar icons. Group members were also given opportunities to examine various leaflets about stroke and aphasia during sessions. Reactions to these were mixed. While some group members felt happy to use one of these booklets to explain their condition to people they met, others did not. Group members rated their own knowledge about stroke and aphasia at the start and end of the term, using pictorial Visual Analogue Scales. These showed an increased level of confidence regarding their own understanding after the project was completed.

The arrival of several new group members the following term, as well as the request from existing members to be reminded of the information they had covered, led the group to extend the project. However, at this stage the group decided to develop the project, with the aim of creating a leaflet to explain stroke and aphasia to other people. There were several advantages to developing a leaflet within the group rather than using one which was already published.

1 The collaborative process of developing the leaflet would in itself provide opportunities for group members to gain and reinforce their understanding of stroke and aphasia.
2 By establishing 'ownership' of the leaflet, group members were able to convey precisely the information that they wished other people to have.
3 The shared and meaningful goal of creating a practical tool for their own use meant that the group (including the new members) quickly became cohesive.

The group worked on the leaflet project for one session a week over a 15-week period, assisted by two student therapists. During the sessions, group members used Total Communication to express their ideas about the information to be included in the leaflet and the format in which it was to be presented. Topics that were selected included general information about stroke and aphasia (see Figure 4.1), their effects, and suggestions of strategies which assist communication (see Figure 4.2). The leaflet included a personalised section for each group member stressing his or her personal strengths. Simple text was written collaboratively between group members and students, and group members produced drawings to convey the information.

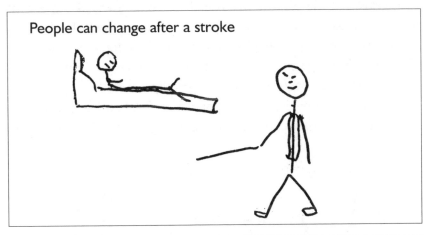

People can change after a stroke

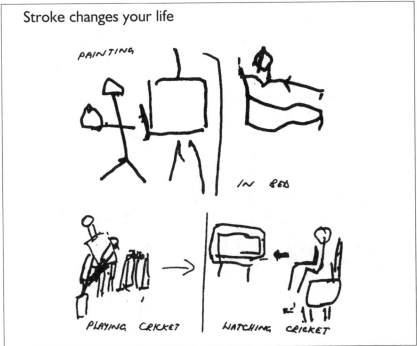

Stroke changes your life

PAINTING

IN BED

PLAYING CRICKET   WATCHING CRICKET

Figure 4.1 *Information about stroke from the stroke and aphasia leaflet project*

The sessions provided opportunities for group members to share their experiences. Sometimes, clients found it painful to reflect on the sudden and traumatic changes they had experienced. At such times group members gave each other support, and maintained consensus that the project was useful to them. Towards the end of the project each client had set a goal to distribute the leaflet beyond the centre. These goals involved identifying the people to whom the leaflet would be given (such as a family member or staff at a day centre) and were recorded pictographically. Once this was carried out, group members reported that the leaflet had been positively received. Graham gave the 'thumbs up' sign, Jim said: 'Oh, lovely' and

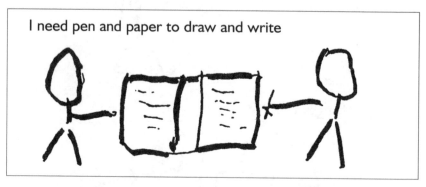

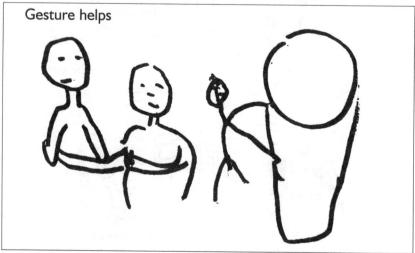

Figure 4.2 *Strategies to assist communication from the stroke and aphasia leaflet project*

Pauline said 'Oh yes, yes'. Jim's wife also relayed her pleasure with the leaflet and reported that Jim's district nurse had asked if she could distribute copies of it to the stroke unit at their local hospital.

Overcoming external barriers: access therapy

Access to information and services seems to be of critical importance for people with aphasia, both in the early stages of stroke and in the long term. People with aphasia have given vivid accounts of struggling with impairment and disability, sometimes for years, unaware of the assistance and services to which they are entitled (Parr *et al*, 1997). Susan's account describes the experience of being unable to obtain essential information which is so common to people with aphasia:

> But ... no nothing ... nothing at all. Just the hospital ... to the hospital then back and nothing only the speech therapy, that's it. But mind I think I don't know. I didn't know it. No services and that. Information of health. Information on money problems. Information on ... rights. (Parr *et al*, 1997, p91)

Such difficulties stem from a number of causes. There is a paucity of information, and very little is accessible to people with aphasia. The information that is available often requires the enquirer to be able to communicate on the telephone or to read complex text, and may be virtually impossible for a person with aphasia to locate in the first place:

> The thing is, I don't know what I'm entitled to – If you don't know where to start you never get nowhere – I don't know. And is not just a matter of scared. (Parr *et al*, 1997, p92)

Such external barriers can be compounded by the lack of confidence in their communication abilities experienced by many people with aphasia, as Alf describes:

> I just couldn't make myself go to ask. It's terrible because you cannot push yourself forward to do these things. (Parr *et al*, 1997, p94)

Access therapy is a type of project work that is specifically focused on overcoming the barriers aphasic clients face in accessing information and services. In addition to the benefits described in the previous section which any project therapy programme may bring, access therapies can have far reaching consequences for client autonomy and community participation. They have been developed in response to the real difficulties that our clients have described, such as getting information about adult education classes that are accessible to people with aphasia, finding out about the range of Social Security benefits to which they may be entitled, or developing the skills and confidence to make use of the facilities available at a local leisure centre.

When aphasic clients wish to obtain information about access to a community service, the most straightforward solution would appear to be for the therapist (or other non-aphasic person) to seek out that information on their behalf and present it to them. Indeed, this should happen if the need for information or service access is urgent or has significant implications for a client's well-being. However, with the client's informed consent, a less urgent need for information can provide a vehicle for a therapy programme which enables the client to develop generalisable strategies as well as the confidence to tackle similar situations which will undoubtedly continue to arise. An aphasia-friendly summary of a group discussion about these issues is presented in Figure 4.3.

While an immediate need can be met in the short term by the therapist taking responsibility, this can have the unintended consequence of maintaining the client's role as a passive recipient. The next time that the client is in the position of needing to obtain information he or she may again feel unable to deal with the situation and rely on the therapist or carer to obtain it, thus perpetuating a dependency which may cyclically undermine the aphasic person's confidence. Clients may also may find themselves in a situation in which they cannot rely on anyone else to assist them (for instance, those with limited support networks) and have no means of obtaining the information or service they require.

It is important to bear in mind that the fundamental aim of access therapy programmes is to promote autonomy through access to information which enables the clients to make informed decisions and take greater charge of the support that they use. This approach to therapy

Goals for the term

- To identify **barriers** that make accessing information about benefits difficult

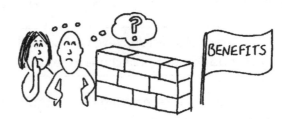

- To identify, develop and practise (at the aphasia centre) alternative approaches and strategies for tackling these barriers

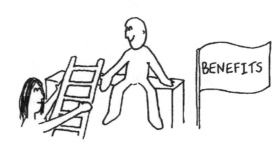

- For all group members to know which benefits they are entitled to

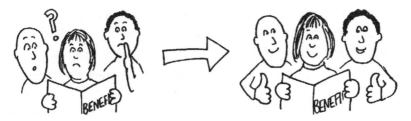

- To feel more confident using the strategies developed in other situations

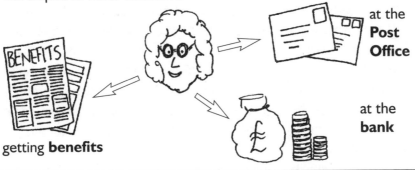

Figure 4.3 *Accessing information and services*

is not about independence in the sense of getting clients to do everything for themselves, but about helping them to know how and where to access information and support. Corbett (1989) comments:

> The basics of self-help, which are second nature to the able-bodied, might be an intolerable chore to some people with disabilities.

Thus, as can be seen from the example of a group access programme described in Case Study 4.2, the enlistment of assistance from other people is promoted as a valid option.

Case Study 4.2 The Citizens' Advice Bureau access project
(The Citizens' Advice Bureau is a network of centres in the UK which provide free advice to individuals about matters such as welfare, finances, statutory and voluntary services and amenities.)

A group of clients who have moderately severe language impairments embarked upon this project, which ran over 10 weekly sessions. The idea for the project arose when Jack, one of the members, told the group that he had just been awarded an additional Social Security benefit that would significantly increase his weekly income. As he had no functional reading skills, severely impaired auditory comprehension and a poor memory, he had been unaware that he might be entitled to this benefit until a friend visiting him from abroad had made enquiries on his behalf. Jack suggested that other members of the group might also be entitled to the same benefit, and that they should apply for it. Group members discussed the benefits that they were each receiving. It quickly became clear that there was considerable variation between individuals and that six of the seven clients felt quite unsure of their entitlement. The group returned to this topic on a number of occasions over the next weeks, prompting the therapist to ask whether the group wished to devote some therapy sessions to finding out what they needed to know – a suggestion that was enthusiastically taken up.

The first step was for the group to set themselves realistic goals and these were agreed after some debate:

- To find out where they might obtain advice about benefits
- To be aware of strategies they might use to assist them in getting information
- To have the opportunity to gain information about their own entitlement to benefits

The therapist and student supported group members in identifying their own solutions to the difficulties of obtaining information. Jack pre-empted this by bringing in a book on pensioners' rights that his friend had used to help him. As none of the group members had sufficient reading skills to permit them to access the information in the book, Jack suggested that the therapist could read it aloud to the group. After some discussion, however, the group vetoed this proposal on the grounds that it would take too much time (the book was more than a hundred pages long) and it was not relevant to everyone (since five of the group members were below retirement age).

With support from the therapist, and using Total Communication, group members spent the next session identifying the nature of the barriers that were preventing them from accessing the information they needed. These included:

- Not knowing where to start in finding out about welfare benefits
- Not being able to understand the leaflets and booklets that contained the necessary information, due to their length and the complexity of the written language
- Being unable to use the statutory benefits advice service dedicated to disabled claimants since this was a telephone helpline, and as such inaccessible to people with marked language impairments

During this session, clients started to use the image of a brick wall to represent the barriers they were encountering (see Figure 4.4). This image was adopted as a standard icon to refer to the concept of barriers throughout the course of therapy.

Over a number of sessions, the group then discussed ways in which they might try to overcome the barriers they had identified.

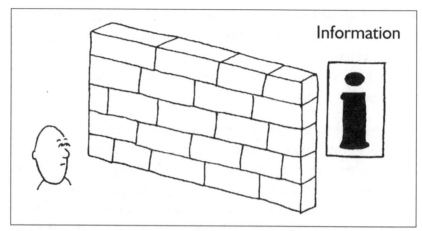

Figure 4.4 *An icon adopted by the group to represent barriers in accessing information*

The therapy progressed at this pace because of the amount of time needed for discussion to take place using Total Communication, and because some group members benefited from frequent repetition of key points.

The first strategy that the group agreed on was to obtain the information in a face-to-face meeting with an advisor, thus avoiding the need to read or use the telephone. One group member, Jennifer, made the suggestion of visiting a Citizens' Advice Bureau. She had done this before, and had found the service useful. The group agreed that this would be a good idea. Discussion followed on how individuals might overcome the barriers to communication they might encounter during a visit to the Citizens' Advice Bureau. While some of the clients felt they could receive assistance from a friend or relative, just as Jennifer had done, others did not have access to such support. The whole group agreed to assist these group members to prepare for their meetings. This preparation took place in two stages.

1 The first stage involved preparing a strategy to explain aphasia to the advisor and convey what assistance was needed in communication. Initially, group members chose to show their wallet-sized cards produced by UK-based charitable bodies, such as The Stroke Association and Action for Dysphasic Adults. These contain a

message to the effect that the bearer has difficulty speaking, reading and writing and asking the other person to speak slowly and clearly. However, the group later rejected this as it was felt that this might not be sufficient guidance if the advisor had never come across anyone with aphasia before. Instead, the group drafted a more detailed explanation with the help of the student therapists.

2 The next stage in planning was to prepare for communicating the details of their enquiry. While some group members felt confident that they could express this effectively and spontaneously using Total Communication, others suggested they would feel more confident if they had some questions prepared on paper beforehand. This was achieved with assistance from the students, and the clients practised asking their questions using role play. One of the group also brought in his benefit payment book to show that this could be used to explain what benefits he was already receiving.

At this stage, the group decided that they were ready to make their appointments at the Citizens' Advice Bureau. They asked one of the students to write a letter explaining their requirements, and Jack used the centre's fax machine to send this to the Bureau located nearby. The reply came the following week. One of the Bureau workers offered to come to the aphasia centre to meet with the whole group and to try to answer their questions. Again, the group nominated the student to make a telephone call to arrange a date for the meeting. The following week, the group discussed how best to use the meeting, since it would be different from the individual appointments they had envisaged. They agreed to ask for some general information about disability benefits that would be relevant to all of them, since there would not be time to discuss their individual circumstances during the one-hour session. With help from the student they modified their written prompts and again, through role play, practised the Total Communication strategies they intended to use.

During this session, the issue of how they might retain the information they were given was raised by a member of the group. They agreed to video record the meeting, with the advisor's consent, so that they could look back at it in future and also share it with other groups. During the meeting, the group successfully asked their questions and received the general information they required. As expected, there was insufficient time for individual entitlements to be discussed in depth, so the advisor put members in touch with the Bureaux which were closest to their own homes.

Evaluation of this therapy programme by group members and the student confirmed that it had been a valuable experience. Although it had taken longer to access the information than it might have done had the therapist simply obtained the relevant leaflets and explained them to the group, the process of finding their own ways to tackle the barriers that they faced had paid other dividends for the group members. They had all become aware of the services of the Citizens' Advice Bureau and recognised that this would be a potential starting point for accessing information in the future. They had also developed communication strategies for accessing information which could again be applied in a range of similar situations. In addition, the fact that all the strategies had been generated by the group members themselves had provided reinforcement of their competence and ability to help themselves and each other. Experiences such as these seem to assist in building confidence and enhancing self-esteem.

Overcoming external barriers: using technology

Technology has featured increasingly in the therapy programmes offered at the centre in recent years. While rarely developed with the needs of disabled people in mind, technology is increasingly providing means by which aphasic people might overcome some of the barriers that they face, particularly with regard to accessing information and participating actively in society. Increasing numbers of people have access to computers and sophisticated telecommunications equipment in the home and work place. While some speech and language therapists have developed innovative ways of utilising technology with their clients (for example, the computer-based therapy developed by the Aphasia Computer Team at Frenchay Hospital, Bristol, UK), others are not always aware of the possibilities that new technologies might offer to their clients, or may not feel confident about using them in therapy due to limited training and experience themselves.

While no-one working at the aphasia centre can claim to be an expert, we have gained some knowledge of technology and telecommunications through trying to find solutions to specific problems identified by individual clients. Technology-based therapy involves a process of jointly identifying the problems to be overcome, problem-solving possible ways around them, seeking out information from other sources and weighing up the available options. Thus it is a process of discovery carried out in partnership which enables clients to find their own technical solutions to overcoming barriers, rather than a situation in which a technical aid is professionally recommended but may end up unused at the back of a cupboard. Some of the technologies which may be useful are described below, but there will undoubtedly be other developments in the near future that will extend the range of tools available to aphasic people. Improvements can also be expected in the systems already available – for instance, through greater accuracy in speech recognition, or improved prosodic modelling in speech synthesis. The suggestions that follow do not of course negate the need for human helpers and advocates. As French (1993) points out, technical aids that are intended to promote independence in disabled people can sometimes be less effective than human assistance. Furthermore, if the use of an aid requires much time or effort on the part of the disabled person this may in fact reduce the opportunities to exercise autonomy over more important aspects of their lives. Therefore technology does not provide the complete solution, and may indeed have a number of drawbacks:

1   Many people, particularly older people who may have had limited experience of using technology, feel anxious or uncomfortable about using machines to accomplish tasks that they could reasonably be helped to do by another person.
2   Depending upon the individual's pattern of language and physical impairments some types of equipment or software may be difficult or impossible to use successfully, since most technology is designed for able-bodied non-aphasic users.

3   Technical aids are often not portable, thus restricting the situations in which they may be used.
4   They can also be prone to breaking down.

Despite these limitations, many people do welcome the possibility of carrying out tasks that they have been unable to do since the onset of aphasia. This can have important implications for autonomy, privacy and self-esteem as well as improving an individual's prospects in a competitive employment market and for accessing educational and leisure opportunities. Some of the uses of computers explored in a recent technology group at the centre are presented in Figure 4.5.

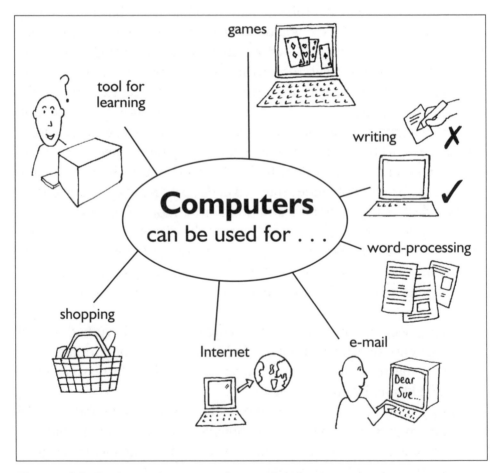

Figure 4.5 *Exploring the potential uses of computers*

The information that follows includes reference to a number of commercially available products. These are given as examples only, and no recommendation of individual products or companies is implied. In a rapidly expanding market new products are often launched, and existing ones updated. For information about new developments in speech and communications technology, try contacting large retailers, specialist communication aid assessment centres or disability advice organisations (such as Abilitynet in the UK).

Technology can make a wide variety of demands on the user's language system. We suggest that a careful assessment of an individual's requirements and abilities is undertaken and specialist advice is sought before any equipment or software is recommended for use by a person with aphasia. Funding might be obtained from charities (such as the Stroke Association Welfare Grants scheme in the UK) and benevolent funds for one-off purchases of equipment, if statutory assistance is not available.

Telecommunications

Many people with aphasia find it much more difficult to communicate by telephone than face to face because communication is restricted to the spoken modality alone. In addition, clients often feel anxious about using the telephone, particularly to speak to strangers. Many avoid making or receiving calls. Relatively low-tech equipment, such as an answerphone that allows you to hear who is calling before picking up the receiver, can often give clients the confidence to answer the telephone at home again. There is also a range of telephones and answerphones that have special features which may help aphasic people to overcome specific difficulties in communicating by telephone.

For instance, Mike had been head of security for an international transport organisation before developing a mild aphasia in his early forties. He planned to return to work in a different professional role, but felt hampered by his difficulty in taking down messages and information over the telephone. Following some enquiries to British Telecommunications Age and Disability Customer Services, we identified a combined telephone and answering machine which could be switched on to record at any time during a telephone conversation. (Telecommunications providers in other countries may be able to offer similar assistance.) This allowed him to record any part of the conversation that he needed to retain and, if necessary, to write the information down later at his own pace. The advent of videophones has also opened up the possibility of people with aphasia using communication strategies such as gesture, drawing and writing during telephone conversations.

Electronic mail systems have also enabled people with relatively intact reading and writing abilities to bypass the need to speak on the telephone in order to have an almost instantaneous exchange of messages with people at a distance, yet to remain unhurried by the immediacy of response required in a telephone conversation.

Case Study 4.3 Aphasia and e-mail: Derek and Jane's stories
Derek was a dentist who, following a stroke, had returned to the UK from Zimbabwe where he had lived for 24 years. He left behind his grown-up daughter and young grandchildren, with whom he now had virtually no contact. As his speech was restricted to a limited number of phrases such as 'I can't read' and 'Come on' and occasional single words, it was impossible for him to keep in touch with his daughter by telephone. He was able to write key words effectively and also to supplement them with drawings using his non-preferred left hand, but was unwilling to send any written communications to his daughter (being somewhat disparaging about his changed writing abilities). Following the purchase of a computer, he asked his therapist about e-mail and requested a demonstration of how it worked on one of the centre's PCs. He quickly learnt how to write and send e-mail messages and began to correspond with his daughter. It was interesting to note that he found his telegraphic style of output acceptable for communicating by e-mail but not in letters.

Another client, Jane, was hoping to return to her job as a political researcher. Because she had mobility difficulties and suffered from fatigue it suited her best to work from home, but this initially seemed impractical because her aphasia made it difficult for her to use the telephone. She was initially uncertain about e-mail, never having used this form of communication before. However, after a period of therapy and with the support of her key worker and another client, she developed the confidence to use it while working from home. She reported that, in addition to the practical benefits it had brought, acquiring these new skills despite her aphasia and mastering a form of modern technology still unfamiliar to many, had given her confidence a much needed boost. Furthermore, developing skills in using e-mail and accessing the internet had also tapped into important identity issues relating to her role as a worker and her skills in conveying information at speed to work colleagues. (For further discussion of identity issues, see Chapter 5.)

Overcoming barriers to writing

Standard word-processing packages incorporate a number of features that can be useful to people with mild to moderate degrees of impairment in written output. Typically, these packages permit multiple revisions to text on screen while still producing a printout of acceptable quality. In addition most packages incorporate automatic spell-checking that highlights any words not recognised by the lexicon and suggests possible near matches, thus aiding correction of orthographic errors even by individuals who are unable to monitor their own writing for mistakes. More sophisticated grammar-check functions can highlight many kinds of sentence construction errors and again suggest acceptable alternatives, although at present these tend to be accessible only to people with mild aphasia.

Some people who make lexical or semantic errors in written output can successfully use on-screen dictionary and thesaurus functions to check their own writing. Although these provide essentially the same information as their printed counterparts, they may be easier to use since they remove the need for the user to scan through pages of alphabetically ordered text. There are also now a number of commercially available software packages which can augment the features found in standard word-processing systems. For example, word prediction programs allow the user to type in the first letter or letters of a word if they cannot access the entire orthographic form. The computer will then suggest a list of the most frequent words beginning with that string from which the user can select the target.

Other programs that can read typed text aloud using text-to-speech synthesis may be useful to those whose self-monitoring of orthographic output is impaired. By setting the program either to read each word aloud as it is typed, or to read a block of text, it becomes possible to identify errors requiring correction that would otherwise have been missed. More recently, applications based on speech recognition software have been developed which may prove of great benefit to people with moderate to severe writing impairments and relatively intact spoken output. Such systems bypass the need to construct orthographic representations by allowing the user to speak directly into a microphone linked to the computer. The program recognises each word and converts it to text which appears on the screen. The text can then be edited (either through speech or keyboard and mouse, depending on which system is being used) and printed or copied to other applications – for example, for sending as an attachment with an e-mail.

Despite their obvious usefulness, such programs do have a number of drawbacks.

- They require an initial time investment both for the user to learn to operate the system and for the system to be trained to recognise the individual user's speech patterns for an extensive database of words.
- They would be of little use to clients who make frequent semantic or phonological errors in their speech or have significant difficulty in constructing sentences.
- Some systems require the spoken input to be segmented by pausing between each word, while more sophisticated systems incorporate mechanisms for segmenting continuous speech into words. Either system will make errors in word recognition and these can be time-consuming to correct.

Rather less high-tech equipment such as tape recorders and dictaphones can also provide practical solutions to functional literacy problems. For example, Sonia had thought for many years about returning to college to retrain as a counsellor as she felt unfulfilled by her current clerical employment. She had not yet applied for any courses as she was concerned that her inability to write quickly would make it impossible for her to take adequate notes. When she discussed this issue with her key worker, they both agreed that this might be overcome if she were permitted to tape record the information she needed. This was proposed to the Disabled Students Officer of the college she hoped to attend, who agreed to arrange this with the tutors.

Overcoming barriers to reading

The difficulties that many people have with reading may also be circumvented to some degree by modern technology. There are a number of ways in which this may be done, most of which involve adapting the presentation of information in a range of formats. Increasingly, information is being produced in a range of formats, including large print and audio cassettes. Although driven primarily by recognition of the needs of those with visual impairments, this can clearly also benefit those aphasic people for whom auditory comprehension is less impaired than reading comprehension. Access to information from newspapers and magazines is also made possible by organisations such as the Talking Newspaper Association in the UK, which provides audio-taped readings of many publications. The principle of access could be further advanced, with personalised information given to a client with reading impairments, perhaps by a therapist, doctor or social worker, on audio tape.

Some people with reading difficulties have found that they are able to access information more easily when it is published in multimedia formats (such as CD-ROM or Internet web pages) which combine text with picture, video and sound images. Input from a therapist may be useful in building confidence in using such formats.

Of course, much information is still produced in text-only formats, and so remains inaccessible to people with reading difficulties, thus placing many restrictions on the type and quantity of information available to them. Another way in which technology may assist aphasic people to overcome this barrier is by converting text into a more accessible form.

Researchers at the universities of Sunderland and Sussex in the UK are currently developing a computer program that will convert complex written text, such as newspaper articles, into a simplified version for aphasic readers (PSET – Practical Simplification of English Text, Devlin & Canning, 1999). It does this in two stages. First, the text is scanned for low frequency vocabulary items and these are replaced with higher frequency synonyms. Second, a syntactic parse is carried out to identify complex sentence structures such as those containing passive verbs or subordinate clauses. These are then converted into simple, canonical structures using the rules of transformational grammar. Although this program is still in development, it may in the future provide a means for making any complex written text more accessible to people with aphasia.

Text can also be made easier to understand by combining it with iconic symbols that emphasise the key points and provide additional semantic information to support language processing. Although it is time consuming to augment written information with symbols by hand, this can be carried out automatically by software programs that can recognise key words in the text and add symbols associated with them.

The technologies just described serve to make text more accessible to people with reading difficulties, but another approach can circumvent the need for the aphasic person to process the written language at all. There are now a number of speech synthesis programs available which can convert text on the computer screen into spoken output. Text can be scanned into the computer and then copied into an application that can produce a synthesised speech output. Although, on current systems, the output sounds rather unnatural and has limited prosodic contours, it nevertheless could provide an aphasic person who has relatively intact auditory processing a means to bypass a damaged reading system and so still gain access to written information.

Case Study 4.4 Using e-mail: Sanjay's story

Sanjay, aged 37, attended the centre once a week for individual therapy. He had studied medicine after leaving school and was due to take up a new post as a junior doctor in a large teaching hospital when he sustained a head injury in a road traffic accident while on holiday. At the time he was 29 years old. The injury resulted initially in a severe cognitive and language processing impairment as well as epilepsy, but left him physically able-bodied. After undergoing a long-term multidisciplinary neuro-rehabilitation programme his impairments had resolved to a moderate level, and he had returned to live at his parents' home.

Sanjay was referred to the centre seven years after his head injury. He lacked confidence and was frustrated by his inability to resume his medical career. Although he had maintained links with many people, he was reliant on his parents to make contact for him since his language impairments meant that he could not effectively communicate by telephone or write letters. He had recently embarked on a vocational rehabilitation programme through which he was employed on a supported work scheme as a catering assistant. His confidence in his own abilities was increasing and he appreciated the opportunities that the work afforded him for communicating with a wider range of people. At the same time, it reinforced the marked fall in his social status when compared to his previous profession. This was an important issue for Sanjay and one that he revisited frequently: 'Me, nine years ago … me doctor.'

Informal assessment of Sanjay's communication showed that he was sociable and made very effective use of his non-verbal communication skills. He still had some cognitive difficulties which affected his ability to maintain relevance within topics of conversation. His turns were often tangential and he frequently related whatever topic was being discussed to one of a narrow range of familiar topics. He had significant auditory comprehension problems. He could usually understand slow speech at a sentence/conversational level, provided there was either a clear context or he was cued in to the topic, but he needed support to maintain his focus. His reading comprehension was more reliable, and auditory comprehension was greatly assisted by the therapist writing key words down and pointing to them to clarify what was being discussed.

Sanjay's own spoken and written output was rather agrammatic, consisting mainly of nouns and short phrases, and he had marked word-finding difficulties. He was always keen to get his message across, and effectively augmented his speech by writing words and phrases and drawing simple diagrams. He had also developed a highly effective strategy of keeping a detailed diary of his activities and contacts, which he would often point to in order to refer to people, places and events.

Sanjay had been attending the centre once a week for three terms before the e-mail therapy programme was started. In therapy, he had focused upon:

- Using communication strategies in a wider range of situations
- Developing his skills and confidence in explaining his communication needs to people in his own environment
- Expanding his social network through joining a badminton club
- Improving his ability to extract core meaning from short texts, and to expand the content and structure of his written output

Sanjay had worked on writing in the context of familiarising himself with some basic computing and word-processing skills that he hoped would expand his employment opportunities. He also worked on developing a personal portfolio, using the centre's word processor, as a way of acknowledging and exploring the profound changes in his personal and social identity (see Chapter 5).

Sanjay purchased a personal computer to allow him to practise his computer skills, and had expressed an interest in learning to access the Internet and to use e-mail. However, he lacked the confidence to try to use his computer at home at all, even to attempt tasks that he was able to carry out on the centre computer.

His key worker therefore visited him at home several times to assist him in transferring his basic word-processing skills to this environment. As he began to feel more confident, Sanjay and his key worker agreed to explore the possibility of his learning to use e-mail. During the first four weeks, sessions were devoted to the following activities:

1 *Supported discussion to establish a shared rationale and aims for the therapy.* This enabled Sanjay to clarify his understanding of how e-mail might assist him to communicate with family and friends, and to identify those people in his environment who had access to e-mail.

2 *Message construction practice.* Attempts to construct a message were more problematic in the context of Sanjay's difficulty: (a)

generating an idea for the e-mail and (b) translating this into some keywords and a construction which would convey his meaning. Together with his key worker, Sanjay clarified the nature of the message he wished to convey, and developed a strategy of writing down a list of keywords related to the subject. He used this written list as a prompt for writing the message, by ordering the keywords and attempting to expand them into phrases. The concept of 'postcard writing' was used to underline the idea that it was not necessary to construct full sentences in an e-mail message (as opposed to the style of writing conventionally employed in letter writing). Sanjay continues to require considerable support in message construction. A further strategy of constructing e-mail 'templates' was used. This was to allow a 'select and copy' approach to writing the e-mail.

3 *Practise sending e-mails.* Sanjay initially sent the messages he had constructed from the centre computer, with his key worker providing both verbal and visual prompts. The visual prompts consisted of step-by-step instructions written in simple phrases which accompanied a printout of the monitor screen as it appears while running the e-mail application. A summary of this step-by-step approach to using e-mail is presented in Figure 4.6. As Sanjay became more familiar with this task, and relied less on the verbal prompts, he took copies of the visual prompts home with him to practise on his own computer. He and his key worker then commenced a weekly e-mail correspondence.

After four sessions, Sanjay had developed a clear understanding of how e-mail might assist him to overcome some of the barriers to communicating with family and friends. He was beginning to be able to construct his own e-mail messages using the keyword strategy, and was able to send and retrieve e-mail messages independently using the visual prompts. He had also acquired basic skills in accessing the Internet to find information – for example, looking up the cricket Test Match scores. He and his key worker therefore agreed to

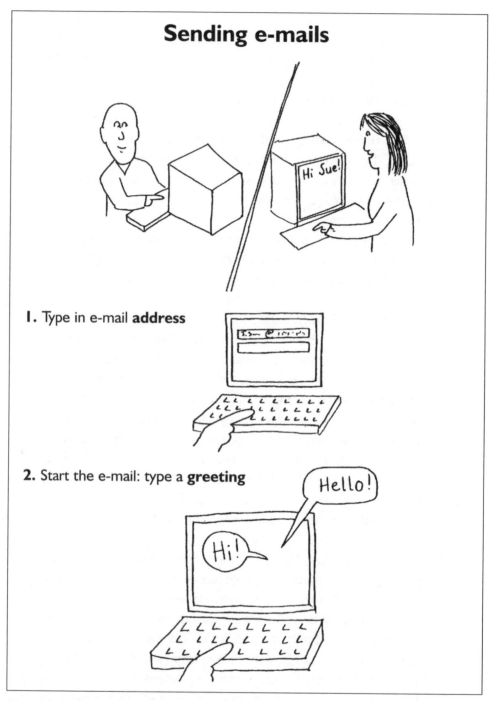

Figure 4.6 *Learning to use e-mail: Sanjay's guide*

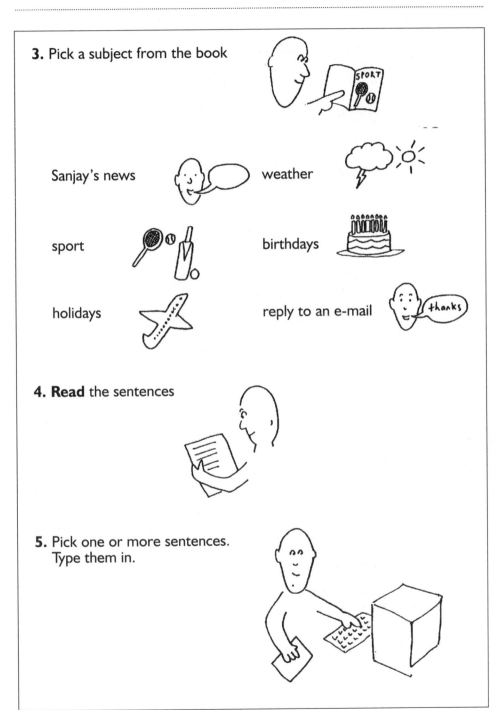

3. Pick a subject from the book

Sanjay's news

weather

sport

birthdays

holidays

reply to an e-mail

4. Read the sentences

5. Pick one or more sentences.
Type them in.

6. End the e-mail: type an **ending**

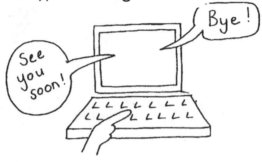

7. Type your **name**

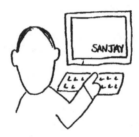

8. Send the e-mail

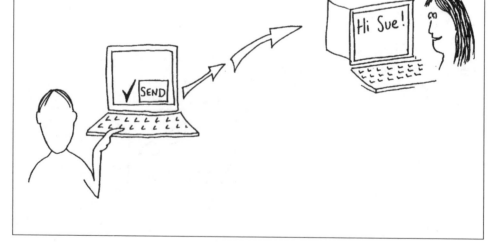

continue this therapy with the aims of consolidating his skills in constructing and using e-mail messages.

This work included more work on developing and utilising e-mail templates. Sanjay's planning and organisational difficulties meant that considerably more input was required on categorising and selecting or amending standard messages. In addition, Sanjay and his father were provided with computer support through similar aphasia-friendly instructions. This was to ensure that Sanjay and his father acquired basic trouble-shooting skills relating to sending and receiving e-mails and that Sanjay's level of success might feed his motivation to keep using the e-mail. It was apparent that Sanjay risked some loss of skill without consistent practice.

Overcoming external barriers: using advocacy

People living with aphasia often have long-term needs for support in accessing social, work and educational opportunities, obtaining information, accessing statutory and voluntary services and managing their own finances and correspondence (Parr *et al*, 1997). In the early stages post-onset, contact with health, rehabilitation and social services may mean that these needs are relatively well provided for (although this is by no means always the case). However, when therapy and rehabilitation ends, many aphasic people are left to negotiate the barriers they encounter without support, with the result that they fail to access essential rights and services. This is particularly true for those clients with moderate or severe aphasia who live alone or for other reasons do not have access to an effective support network. One way of providing aphasic people with support to overcome the societal barriers that they face, while retaining their autonomy, is through advocacy.

What is advocacy?

Essentially, it means that one individual acts on behalf of another who may have difficulty participating in society and/or exercising their rights. An advocate will usually act as a supporter or enabler, but may, where necessary, clarify information or speak on the other person's behalf in order to represent that person's point of view:

> Advocacy... requires an active commitment to represent another's interests as if they were your own. (Tyne, 1994, p250)

While people with aphasia have always used the support of informal advocates (such as caregivers), more formal advocacy has tended to be associated with other groups such as people with learning disabilities or mental health needs. A formal advocate can offer a combination of autonomy and support, and this has obvious relevance for people with aphasia:

> Regaining mastery over their own situation through informed decision making is an important step for clients in both their rehabilitation and empowerment. (Maclaren, 1996, p497)

Advocacy can take many forms, including:

- Informal support from family and friends – for example, with reading and writing letters
- Professional advocacy provided, for instance, by a speech and language therapist or lawyer for a limited period and usually in relation to a particular issue
- Long-term advocacy partnerships, usually provided on a voluntary basis, to assist individuals to participate in their community and exercise their rights

The decision to set up long-term advocacy is often taken when a client is preparing to leave the centre. Although client and therapist may agree that the client can no longer benefit from active therapy, well founded anxieties often surface about how the client will cope without the support that they have, until this point, received at the centre (such as assistance in filling in forms and reading important letters). In settings where therapeutic time and input is limited by restricted resources or prescriptive service contracting, accessing and training an advocate to support an aphasic individual in the long term may, for some individuals, provide greater benefit than a brief programme of impairment-focused therapy.

Finding an advocate

In many cases, support will come from a family member or friend whom the client already knows and trusts. It may be helpful for the therapist to facilitate a dialogue between this person and the client to establish what sort of assistance the client does and does not require. It is important to be explicit at this stage; otherwise the friend or relative may, with the best of intentions, take on an overly protective role, and promote dependency rather than autonomy. However, it is equally important not to disrupt the balance of a multifaceted relationship that works for the individuals involved. As far as possible, client and advocate should be facilitated to find their own solutions to problems encountered. This may be difficult if:

- the delicate balance of a relationship cannot easily accommodate advocacy
- either member of the dyad feels unable to develop an advocacy relationship
- the client lives alone and has a limited support network
- the client's need for privacy makes it inappropriate for a close associate to assist him or her in this role

In such situations, it becomes necessary to try to identify an individual whose primary relationship with the aphasic person can centre on his or her role as advocate.

Therapists should not underestimate the difficulties they may encounter when trying to find an advocate for an aphasic client. Ideally, advocates can be found through existing advocacy services in voluntary and statutory sectors. Advocates from these sources should have received training in advocacy skills, and should have access to ongoing support and supervision in fulfilling their role. However, provision of advocacy services is patchy and, in most cases, services specify criteria for who is eligible to use them. For instance, services may exist in some areas only for adults with learning disabilities, for refugees and for those experiencing mental health problems, but not for people with other needs.

The exclusion of people with communication impairments by advocacy services can sometimes be explicit. Some services:

> cannot match advocates with people who have no voice, or no clear way of expressing their wishes. So some of those people who are likely to have the very greatest need for a way of protecting their interest may be denied advocacy. (Tyne, 1994, p251)

However, our experience has shown that it may be possible to overcome these barriers provided the therapist is willing to take on the role of advocate for the client in the first instance, in order to facilitate access to an advocacy service. Through persistent explanation of aphasia and individual needs, we have found that individual service coordinators may be prepared to adopt a more flexible approach and take on an aphasic client. Although this process can be time-consuming, it can alert existing services to the fact that there is a significant unmet need.

If, after exploring all the possible advocacy services in the local area, advocacy support for a client has not been found, it may be possible to arrange this on a more ad hoc basis – for instance, through a local volunteer bureau or church. In this situation, it is important that the therapist provides some ongoing support to the advocate, at least in the early stages, to enable them to meet the needs of the aphasic person effectively. Whatever the source of the advocate, the speech and language therapist has an important role to play in training them to understand their client's impairments, and to use strategies which effectively support communication.

Case Study 4.5 Aphasia and advocacy: Steve's story

At 35, Steve had an intra-cerebral haemorrhage which left him with moderately severe aphasia, but no major physical impairments. He attended the centre for three years. Steve had been married with three young children, although after the stroke his marriage had broken up and he had lived alone since then. He spent several long vacations each year with his elderly mother in Devon, who was also his main source of support in managing his affairs and correspondence. This was achieved by Steve forwarding all his post directly to his mother who would deal with it on his behalf. Although she was happy to provide this support to Steve, his mother felt that it would be better for him to have assistance locally. She felt that his return to dependence on her during adult life was continually undermining his self-esteem. She also knew that Steve would have to cope without her at some stage in the future. Steve had become fairly isolated from his pre-stroke friends, due in part to his embarrassment at his communication difficulties.

Previously self-employed as a plumber, Steve had been out of work since his stroke. His only income was from state disability benefits. Two years after his stroke, Steve had attended a rehabilitation/employment assessment course. This had concluded that his manual and technical skills were at a high level and that he should be able to return to skilled work in an environment where he was given assistance with communication and following instructions. However, he had never felt confident enough to attempt this, in light of the competitive nature of the job market. Steve decided that he would be unable to return to self-employment. The possibility of voluntary work had begun to appeal to him as it might provide a stepping stone back into paid work.

During his first two years at the centre, individual therapy focused largely on his language impairments (working on semantic categorisation, expanding use of adjectives in spoken output, developing phoneme-to-grapheme conversion skills, and practising auditory comprehension of spoken passages) while group sessions encouraged the use of Total Communication. At the beginning of his third year at the centre, it was apparent that his language impairments had remained stable for some time and that, while he was able to employ a range of communication strategies when prompted during therapy sessions, there had been only limited carryover to other situations. It was also clear that Steve still hoped therapy would 'cure' him of his impairments and was frustrated by the limited progress he had made. Both Steve and his therapist acknowledged that the main benefit that he now derived from attending the centre was regular social contact and support. They decided to shift the focus of intervention away from impairment-level therapies on to looking at the impact of Steve's aphasia on his lifestyle and aspirations.

Individual therapy sessions were spent discussing Steve's current opportunities and needs in relation to social, leisure and occupational aspects of his lifestyle, as well as facilitating him to clarify his personal aims for the future. These discussions created the opportunity for Steve and his therapist openly to discuss his prognosis for further change in his language and communication skills, and Steve began to adjust his expectations of therapy. It was agreed that preparations should be made for him to leave therapy.

Steve made it clear that he would feel ready to leave the centre if he could find suitable employment that would give him regular opportunities for social contact, but that he was anxious about his ability to cope on his own. A major concern was that he would become bored and isolated once he left the group since this had provided his main social contact for several years. He felt that this would be overcome if he could find work (paid or voluntary) which would give him opportunities to mix with a wider group of people. He felt that he would need support to find and apply for suitable work: to understand job advertisements, complete application forms and communicate at interviews. Steve also echoed at this time his mother's concerns about his dependence on her for help in managing his affairs. He did not feel his local self-help group would provide all the assistance he needed in this and in reinvolving himself in his local community.

Steve and his therapist therefore negotiated a plan to assist him to move on from attending regular therapy sessions into a more long-term support network. They decided to obtain information about advocacy services available in Steve's local community, to investigate the availability of training courses and employment opportunities in conjunction with Steve's local Disability Employment Advice service, and to explore the possibility of voluntary employment through his local volunteer bureau.

The first step in trying to find an advocate for Steve was to contact the information services provided by Citizen Advocacy Information and Training and by a local disability advice centre. This revealed that there was an established service in the area, but that it was designated for adults with learning difficulties.

The therapist contacted this service to outline Steve's advocacy needs and the organiser agreed to some tentative contact. The therapist and key worker then drafted information about Steve's aphasia and strategies that assisted him to communicate, as well as a report describing his social situation and the type of assistance he might need from an advocate. Steve, his key worker and Karen (the advocacy organiser) met to discuss the situation. All felt that the meeting went well and agreed to pursue the idea of finding an advocate for Steve. Karen explained that it sometimes took time to match an individual with a suitable advocacy partner, but that in the meantime she would keep in touch with him (for instance, by going out together for coffee) in order to provide him with access to support and to keep him informed of progress. She also offered to apply on Steve's behalf to a local charity for funding for a driving reassessment that he was keen to undertake. Karen demonstrated very effective facilitation skills during the meeting and did not require any further training in this area.

During the same period, Steve's key worker accompanied him to a meeting at the local volunteer bureau. A number of opportunities for volunteering were offered to him, including joining an environmental conservation group and carrying out maintenance at a local zoo. Steve accepted the job at the zoo as this would mean working alongside other people in an interesting environment and because he could make use of his considerable practical skills and experience. He left the aphasia centre.

Karen maintained her contact with Steve while she tried, unsuccessfully, to find a him a suitable advocate. She was a valuable source of support during his transition to life beyond the centre. Finally, Karen offered to be his long-term advocacy partner herself. Her support included accompanying him into situations in which he did not feel confident about his communication skills, assisting him with correspondence and telephone calls and helping him to access a wide range of information and services. This partnership has been maintained for over two years and has provided the confidence that Steve needs to cope with life with aphasia, while not compromising his autonomy.

Overcoming internal barriers: stress management and assertiveness

Stress management

There are a number of reasons why stress management is useful in aphasia therapy. People with aphasia often experience high levels of stress, both in the early stages of aphasia and in the long term as they deal with the consequences of their impairments. The frustration of experiencing communication breakdown on a daily basis cannot be underestimated, and has been well documented in the literature (for example, Friedman, 1961; Bardach, 1969; Benson, 1980; Ricco-Schwartz, 1980). In addition to the stresses that accompany impaired communication, people with aphasia often experience major, unforeseen life changes, difficulties in maintaining personal relationships and loss of personal autonomy.

Communication and physical impairments may compromise many of the strategies that an individual might previously have used to relieve stress. It may be difficult, for example, to talk problems over with a friend, to pursue an interest, or to relax by reading, watching television, or taking physical exercise. Many forms of professional support (such as counselling or traditional stress management groups) are inaccessible to people with aphasia because of their reliance on sophisticated verbal communication.

There seems to be a strong link between emotional state and communication abilities. Most people will agree that their abilities to take in information or express themselves deteriorate when they are anxious or distressed, and this trait appears to be increased in people with aphasia. Aphasic clients often do less well in language assessments if they are highly anxious about the test situation, and it is common for communication strategies which can be used effectively in a supportive therapy session to break down when the client is faced with the stress of a difficult situation in real life.

It seems likely, therefore, that the effectiveness and generalisation of language and communication-focused therapies may be enhanced by the integration of stress management techniques (Julia Richey, personal communication, 1994). With the health implications of stress being increasingly recognised, stress management can also play a role in health promotion for our clients. Stress management can be incorporated into aphasia therapy explicitly as a programme in its own right, or be integrated implicitly into work on language and communication, both with individual clients and in groupwork. Case Study 4.6 illustrates how a stress management approach was implemented with a group of clients with aphasia.

Case Study 4.6 Dealing with difficulties: the Stress Management Group

This group was run at a West Lambeth Community Care NHS Trust community health centre. The group was made up of eight men and two women, aged between 32 and 81 years, with the average time since onset of aphasia being 21 months. All the group members had mild/moderate impairments of auditory comprehension, and were able to follow a group discussion with limited support. (However, similar groupwork at the centre has also been effective with people who have severe comprehension impairments.) Impairments of spoken and written expression ranged from minimal to severe. Reasons for joining the stress management group varied, but all group members acknowledged the stress of living with aphasia and wished to find new ways to cope with the difficulties they faced with others 'in the same boat'.

Group members were in very different living situations and had different experience of living with aphasia. For example, Mark was an electrician who had been aphasic for nine months and lived with his wife. He had a mild fluent aphasia and was skilled at using a range of strategies to compensate for his word-finding and auditory processing difficulties. He was confident about communicating in most situations, but had become very anxious about speaking to strangers on the telephone. This was restricting his ability to obtain work. Frank was a retired priest. His stroke had resulted in problems with mobility and personal care, and he now lived in a residential care home. His speech and auditory comprehension were only slightly affected, but he had more marked difficulties reading and writing. Frank had found it very difficult to adjust to the change in his communication particularly since his vocation had depended so much on his effective interpersonal skills. He had now become very anxious about communicating and was aware that he found it more difficult to process language when he was feeling stressed. Felicity, 67, was a retired statistician. She had never married and lived with her younger sister. A stroke had resulted in an almost total loss of speech. She had come to rely on writing as her main mode of expression but her messages were often unclear due to semantic errors and paragrammatic sentence construction. Her auditory and reading comprehension was relatively intact, and she was very frustrated by her inability to speak. She had found that many of the leisure activities she had previously enjoyed were now difficult, and she had been unable to resume her work as a volunteer in the office of a large charity. A fiercely independent woman, she was also distressed by her changed role at home since she now relied on her sister to communicate for her in many situations.

The group met once a week for one and a half hours over a 10-week period. Sessions were facilitated by two speech and language therapists (who were joined for one session by Harry Clarke, the centre's counsellor). The general purpose of the group was to reduce perceived levels of stress among group members, and this was broken down into a number of aims:

- To identify common and individual sources of stress
- To explore the stress of communication breakdown
- To identify personal responses to stress (physical, behavioural, cognitive and emotional)
- To identify personal styles of coping with stress
- To expand individual repertoires of coping strategies
- To gain experience in the use of a range of relaxation techniques
- To reduce anxiety about stroke illness through receiving accurate and accessible information
- To develop long-term support networks.
  (Aims adapted from Julia Richey, personal communication, 1994.)

The group engaged in a wide range of activities. Some of these focused on more general aspects of stress which all people experience as they negotiate the ups and downs of life, while others were specifically focused on issues related to aphasia and communication breakdown. An ongoing challenge throughout the therapy programme was for the therapists to ensure that activities and discussions were accessible to all members of the group despite their varying language and communication difficulties. Tasks were therefore adapted to allow participation through Total Communication, and the therapists ensured that all the clients were given access to the floor in order to share their ideas and experiences. Some examples of activities are described below.

Group brainstorming
One session was spent collectively identifying some of the physical symptoms of stress. Each client was provided with a sheet of paper on which was drawn a blank, generic human shape, plus pens and pencils. Each person was asked to use this image to show one or more symptoms that they might experience when they were feeling stressed. Group members had time to think about the task, and to draw or write their ideas on the paper. Each person then fed back his or her contribution to the whole group by showing the sheet of paper. Drawn messages were often expanded using pointing, gesture, facial expression and speech. The therapist collated all the contributions onto the flipchart, resulting in the summary shown in Figure 4.7.

There were two reasons for doing this. One was to raise awareness of 'warning signs' so that group members would quickly recognise when stress levels were rising and a stress management technique might be useful. The other was to provide a basis for a later discussion on health and stress.

Information giving
Using keywords and drawings on an overhead projector, the therapist illustrated the stress symptoms identified by the group, in terms of the 'fight or flight' response. The factors contributing to hypertension and atherosclerosis were outlined, and their relationship to stroke illness described. The group went on to discuss

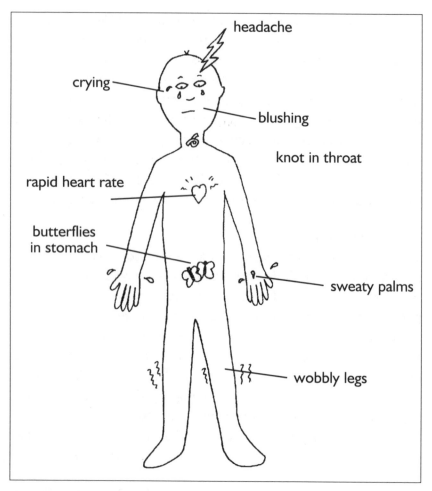

Figure 4.7 *The impact of stress*

a number of strategies they could use, in addition to taking prescribed medication, in order to promote a healthier lifestyle and cut down the risk of stroke. These included measures such as cutting down on smoking, reducing salt intake, maintaining a healthy weight, relaxing and taking regular exercise.

Using drawing to explore emotional responses
Group members were encouraged to reflect upon and discuss the emotional impact of stress. Drawing was used as a medium of discussion, so that it would be accessible to all group members

regardless of their language skills. Once paper, pens, pencils and coloured crayons had been given out, the therapist asked the group to think how it felt to be stressed and how it felt to be calm, then to draw these different states. The therapist gave some examples using her own drawings. Group members could do the task in any way they wished, using abstract or concrete images and a range of colours (see Figure 4.8). All but one of the group members (who felt uncomfortable using non-verbal means of expression) enjoyed this task and wished to share their pictures with the whole group. It was found to be an effective way of conveying abstract concepts without reliance on language, and led to a supportive group discussion on the emotional impact of aphasia.

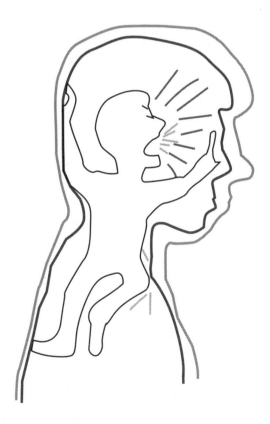

Figure 4.8 *Daniel's drawing to represent stress and aphasia*

Relaxation techniques
The group members indicated that they wished to learn how to relax. Their pictures of stressed and calm states were used to introduce three possible relaxation techniques which they could use. These were:

- Progressive muscular relaxation (using a commercially available tape)
- A diaphragmatic breathing exercise
- Guided visualisation while listening to relaxing music.

These techniques, once introduced and tried out, were then discussed. A number of alternative techniques such as yoga, massage and aromatherapy were also discussed, but not tried out.

Story boards and role play
Individual styles of response to stressful situations were explored through story boards. In this activity, each person is given a sheet of paper divided into four boxes. In the first box, they are asked to draw a character (which may be a simple stick figure, an abstract shape, or a detailed sketch). In the second box, clients are asked to draw a stressful situation in which the character finds himself. In the third box, clients draw how the character feels about the situation. In the final box, they depict what he does next. Story boarding is useful in allowing clients to reflect upon personal coping styles in a 'safe' way, since it is the character and not themselves whom they are describing. Role play was also used to explore strategies for dealing with stressful situations, and this gave an opportunity for clients to try out new strategies in a safe and supportive environment, and to evaluate their effectiveness.

Practising stress management strategies in real-life situations
Having tried out various techniques at the centre, clients were encouraged to put them into practice outside the group. The group was encouraged to set realistic, achievable goals at this point. Some were carried out during the sessions (such as approaching a passer-by in the street outside the centre to ask for directions) and others at home (such

as relaxing before making a phone call). Group feedback allowed for further discussion, sharing of good and bad experiences, and identification of alternative strategies when things had not gone well.

Evaluation

It is not easy to specify the effects of a course of stress management therapy. This is because it may contribute to changes on a number of different parameters including self-confidence and esteem, functional communication, lifestyle, knowledge about stress and stroke, establishment of supportive relationships and use of relaxation techniques. In addition, many changes will be subtle and may continue to accumulate long after therapy has ended. Nevertheless, the stress management course was evaluated using qualitative methods, such as group discussion and some individual interviews, through a survey of client satisfaction, and with a communication stress questionnaire that was devised for the purpose. All these evaluation methods indicated that positive changes had taken place, and that the clients were dealing more effectively with their stress.

Assertiveness training

To be assertive means positively claiming one's rights or defending one's opinions in a manner that is respectful of the rights and opinions of others. Assertiveness is a way of thinking, behaving and communicating that differs from both passivity and aggression, either of which can stem from low self-esteem:

> The key to assertive behaviour is feeling good about ourselves ... Assertive behaviour ... results in a feeling of inner strength and enables us to take control of our lives. (Holland & Ward, 1990, p5)

The imbalance of control over interaction that can result from the linguistic impairment of aphasia can make it difficult for aphasic people to make their thoughts, opinions and wishes known. It may become difficult to exercise autonomy on a number of levels, whether in the course of a social chat or through involvement in major life decisions.

As discussed in Chapter 1, people with aphasia are often disabled by the negative attitudes and reactions of those around them. This issue is discussed by Kagan in terms of 'masking of competence':

> When a person has difficulty in talking and understanding what is said, it is difficult to 'see' the active mind; it is difficult to envisage the capacity to make life decisions; and it is difficult to regard the person as a social being. These perceptions affect the way one is treated. (Kagan, 1995, p17)

Negative attitudes are stigmatising, and make it even more difficult for people with aphasia to engage in interactions on an equal footing with others. In addition, people with aphasia may have internalised the negative perceptions of communication impairment which are prevalent in society. They may lack self-esteem and confidence in their own communication abilities (Wahrborg & Borenstein, 1988; D'Afflitti & Weitz, 1974). These factors can compound the experience of communication disability, contributing to a sense of powerlessness in interactions with other people. While it is necessary, in the long term, to address attitudinal barriers at a societal level (for instance, through media representation that raises awareness of communication impairment), such change is difficult to effect and tends to occur slowly, if at all. Part of the role of the therapist is therefore to support people with aphasia in developing the personal resources, skills and confidence with which to counter the prejudice and inequality that they face on a daily basis.

People with aphasia can to some degree compensate for impaired language skills and counter the negative reactions of others through adopting an assertive style of communication. The ability to be assertive does not necessarily correlate with the degree of language impairment an individual has. Rather, as Holland and Ward (1990) point out, assertive communication depends upon a number of factors:

- Belief in one's own rights
- Respect for the rights of others
- Good listening skills

- Expression of thoughts and feelings
- Use of non-verbal communication skills

There are many practical guides on the topic of assertiveness (for example, Holland & Ward, 1990). Many of the activities suggested here are drawn from these, but have been adapted to meet the requirements of our clients – for example, through the use of Total Communication and through the explicit focus on issues relating to aphasia. Assertiveness training can be incorporated into individual therapy, but a supportive group environment is often very helpful.

Activities involved in assertiveness work

Discussion to clarify the meaning of assertiveness and attitudes towards it

Assertiveness is an abstract concept which may elude clear definition and discussion, particularly by people who have severely impaired language. The concept can be made more accessible through:

- Role play by the therapist illustrating assertive, aggressive and passive styles of communication.
- Short clips on video showing people communicating or behaving in ways which are clearly assertive or non-assertive.
- Iconic representations of assertive and other styles of communication which can be used to support discussion.
- Brainstorming to establish a 'Bill of Rights' in communication, which might include:

  1 The right to be listened to
  2 The right to have time to express myself
  3 The right to make up my own mind
  4 The right to be given information in ways that I can understand

Once established, group members and therapists might agree to uphold the Bill of Rights in their interactions with each other, thus encouraging a sharing of responsibility for communication and participation in the group. The concept of personal rights also underpins sessions relating to assertive communication in situations outside the centre.

- Identifying those aspects of communication and behaviour which make up assertive, aggressive and passive styles. These might include features such as eye contact, facial expression, gesture, body posture, proximity between people, voice quality, intonation, loudness of speech and use of vocabulary. Again it can be useful for group members to observe role play or video-taped interactions in order to identify specific features of behaviour.

Personal experiences of difficult communication situations
Group discussion can be used to explore the issue of when it might be more appropriate to adopt assertive, aggressive or passive styles of communication, and to acknowledge personal preferences in communication style.

How does communication style influence the outcome of an interaction?
This issue can be explored through discussion of group members' own experiences, story board drawing and role play. Using pictorial or key word checklists, group members identify the styles of communication used by individuals in a particular situation. They consider the extent to which those individuals achieved their aims in the interaction and how the outcome might impact on their confidence and self-esteem.

Experimenting with styles of communication
Group members adapt features (such as body posture and intonation) which have been identified as a component of assertive and non-assertive behaviour. This can be done through role-playing situations using different communication styles, listening to feedback, practising strategies in more natural interactions within the group, and trying out different styles in real-life situations that arise.

Evaluation

The outcomes of assertiveness work are not easy to evaluate since they can effect changes that are often subtle, and that operate on a range of parameters. Some of the benefits that we have observed include:

- Increased confidence in communication, demonstrated both through self-rating scales and in observable changes in communication style.
- Increased awareness of and commitment to equality in communication, as demonstrated by changed group dynamics. For example, one group was heavily dominated by a single group member whose style of communication was at times aggressive, while two of the other group members took virtually no turns during discussions. By the end of the term's work this pattern had changed significantly. The quieter members started to initiate some major turns and persisted in stating their opinions when negated or misunderstood by other group members. The dominant group member still played an active role, while creating conversational openings and encouragement for others to participate. These changes were captured on video at different stages in the therapy process.

Clients have evaluated changes in communication style themselves, using checklists of communication features to analyse each other's contributions in video-taped discussions. Individual goals related to assertiveness have also proved useful for evaluating how far clients have been able to put their skills into practice in real-life situations. These have often been linked to communication opportunities arising through other therapy such as access and project work, as well as to situations arising naturally in clients' own environments.

Probably the most subtle aspect of assertiveness work (and the most difficult to evaluate) concerns its contribution to the development of a personal identity which accommodates the changes associated with communication impairment. This complex issue, and some of the therapies that might be useful in supporting the development of a robust, disabled identity, will be described in Chapter 5.

CHAPTER 5

Developing Therapies for Developing Identities

The real me is before the stroke ... now is nothing. (Paul)

What is identity?

It has long been recognised that aphasia has a major impact on a person's sense of self and that the concern with personal adaptation forms a crucial part of the therapeutic endeavour (Brumfitt, 1993; Gainotti, 1997). As Sarno (1997) comments:

Finding a new identity, as a member of a community of chronically disabled individuals is a crucial component of the aphasic person's reaching an acceptable and positive level of life satisfaction. Since the sense of belonging usually requires the experience of feeling social approval, this presents a special challenge to the person with aphasia. (Sarno, 1997, p676)

In the past, however, therapists have perhaps been less than clear in describing the ways in which they address this complex issue in therapy, and evidence suggests that it may indeed be somewhat neglected (Parr *et al*, 1997). Reasons for this might include the time constraints on contracts of care, an explicit focus of input on the rehabilitation of communication, and feelings of inadequacy experienced by therapists when faced with life issues rather than communication skills.

As described in Chapter 1, identity is one of the key concerns of social model thinking (Peters, 1999). To simplify this somewhat, at least three types of identity are discernible. *Personal identity* concerns the development, establishment and maintenance of a person's sense of self, the personal biography. There is increasing interest in illness as 'biographical disruption' (Bury, 1991) and in exploring identity changes brought about by illness, using narrative methods (Frank, 1995). *Social identity* refers to the individual being part of (or excluded from) various social and cultural groups, communities and institutions (Corker, 1996). *Collective identity* refers to the sense of group unity, parity and action that is often the hallmark of political and pressure groups, and in which individual concerns are, to a certain extent, subsumed.

At the aphasia centre, we aim to support the individual in re-establishing and maintaining robust personal, social and collective identities in the aftermath of impairment. Clearly, this will mean different things to different people but, in the context of aphasia, it refers to living a life in which language impairment is a part of the big picture – not an insignificant part, or one which is not an ongoing cause of struggle and frustration – but a part that is integrated into the whole of a person's life.

Inevitably, the therapist who aims to support the client in dealing with the disruption of suddenly acquired impairment will need to draw heavily on counselling and listening skills. We are fortunate to have the service of two trained counsellors (who have personal experience of aphasia) at the centre. However, in this chapter, rather than addressing the counselling process which is already well documented (for example, in Syder, 1998), we aim to describe therapeutic approaches which move beyond traditional counselling methods. These explicitly focus on issues of identity by fostering self-exploration, self-actualisation and personal growth.

Before presenting some ideas for identity-focused therapies, it is perhaps important to make the point that identity issues are not just relevant to the person with aphasia. They also shape the aphasia therapist (influencing therapeutic beliefs and practice) and, indeed, characterise the institution or organisation in which therapy is delivered. In the remainder of this introductory section, we start to unpick the tangle of issues around personal, social and collective identities for these three entities – the person with aphasia, the therapist and the organisation – by looking at illness beliefs and reflexivity, roles and partnership, power and expertise, and the use of positive role models.

Illness beliefs and reflexivity

The person with aphasia comes to therapy with an established set of personal health beliefs and a range of strategies and styles for dealing with illness and loss (Kleinman, 1988; Frank, 1995). These may be rooted in familial, cultural or personal experiences but, whatever their origins, they undoubtedly impact on the individual's way of coping with the differences now faced. Therapists may choose to work within or around these influences, and are hopefully aware that such factors have a critical impact upon a person's response to therapy.

Accessing beliefs and attitudes that are implicit and may be rarely articulated is no straightforward matter, whether or not aphasia is present. The process of learning about a person's understanding of illness and impairment and hearing his or her story must inevitably involve skilled interviewing and intensive listening. If possible, this should adhere to the person's own chronology of events and developments, moving away from therapeutic constructs and beyond the usual case-history format. Another important part of this process concerns the awareness and personal reflection of the therapist/facilitator regarding his or her own understanding of disability.

Therapist and client may have a very different understanding of what it means to live with aphasia. In a study comparing the beliefs and attitudes regarding language impairment of people with aphasia and therapists, Pound (1993) found a striking level of dissonance. One of the key points of disagreement concerned the overwhelmingly negative outlook of therapists regarding life after stroke. Speech and language therapists focused almost exclusively on what they viewed as the inevitably destructive impact of impaired communication. This was not the case for a number of the aphasic people interviewed, who identified both positive and negative factors in their new life with aphasia. It was clear, too, that for people with aphasia, language impairment may be only one of a number of other major life issues following the onset of stroke. Other considerations, such as being much slower at completing routine activities, not having a job, or being unable to drive, were deemed as important as communication issues, whereas the latter were often the therapists' key and even sole concern. This evidence accords with the findings from a qualitative study of the subjective experience of aphasia (Parr *et al*, 1997) and a study of self-advocacy in aphasia (Penman, 1998).

Gaining the confidence to broaden out from concern with communication impairment and pay attention to the individual's personal story is not easy. Inevitably, therapists bring their own models to such an endeavour, shaped by personal experience, training, and the work setting and ethos. Fortunately, many training courses and initiatives in support and supervision now encourage therapists to enter a period of critical reflection and to develop a reflective approach to what they do. Therapists are increasingly aware of the power of dominant discourses and the modernist constructions of illness and cure that have underpinned traditional approaches to rehabilitation (Frank, 1995; Barrow, 1999).

Unless clinicians have at least some grasp on their personal views on competence and disability and the way these influence their therapeutic interactions, the potential for disempowerment and dependency in therapy will be a constant threat. There is no easy recipe for true empowerment. Parsloe and Stevenson (1993) comment:

> The self-awareness of workers is crucial so that they can be aware of excessive anxiety and over-protectiveness or of the hidden satisfaction which they derive from the benign exercise of power. Such an insight is not a luxury, it is a necessity if processes of empowerment are to be effective. (Parsloe & Stevenson, 1993, p21)

Roles and partnerships
The health professional first encounters the person with aphasia frozen in a post brain-injury snapshot and, unless great care is taken, stripped of context, biography and belief. The 'patient' enters rehabilitative and

therapeutic rituals and may indeed be defined and regarded in terms of the nature of his or her impairment. How often have you heard a health professional say: 'I've got a fluent aphasic' or 'We have two new dysphasics on the ward'? Given the threat to existing roles and the uncertainties of sudden illness, it is hardly surprising if a person with aphasia readily assumes and fiercely maintains the role of patient, particularly when in a hospital context.

The 'patient role' is underpinned by a number of assumptions: the desire to get better; the belief that this will happen; the expectation that doctors and therapists are there to make this happen and that the patient must cooperate with them and work hard (Parsons, 1967). These assumptions are shaped by what Frank (1995) has called the 'restitution narrative' which forms the basis of modernist medical practice. The restitution narrative arises from the expectation that medicine (or other powers) can and will get you better. Within this structure, doctors and therapists are expert and often heroic fixers, and patients the tragic or long-suffering victims waiting to be rescued from their afflictions.

These values imbue hospitals and rehabilitation facilities, influencing those who give and receive medical care. They are affirmed and reaffirmed in media representations of illness and disability and in popular culture to powerful effect (Barnes, 1996; French, 1994). The expert role, which many therapists assume or have thrust upon them, is also much represented and often glamorised, supported in drama, newspaper articles, advertisements, documentaries and other forms of media, and evident most notably in stories of the marvel of science and breakthrough cures. Therapists working within a social model approach need to understand the allure of the restitution culture and develop new identities in relation to the person with aphasia.

Power and expertise

> I had so much trust and respect for her ... if she'd told me jumping off a bridge into the water would help my speech ... I'd have done it.

This quotation from a person with aphasia (cited in Pound, 1993) illustrates a degree of confidence in a therapist's expertise which is both alarming and, to be honest, alluring. It highlights the many difficulties that may arise when a therapist attempts to move away from traditional identities and to convince the person with aphasia that they too have an expert role to play in what is essentially a therapeutic partnership. However, professional expertise is hard won, and the power which accompanies it is sometimes reluctantly yielded or shared.

Expertise may be gathered through experience, training, contact and debate with colleagues, challenge from those within and outside the profession, the hard work of learning, the pressure of doing and time for reflection. Opportunities to do this are often available to the therapist, and should be extended to people with aphasia. A first step must be the explicit acknowledgement of the person's intrinsic competence along with delineation of what the therapist can and cannot offer. Sharing power and expertise and developing a true partnership between therapist and client may be a tortuous process, fraught with obstacles – fluctuations in confidence, exacerbations of illness and fatigue, disempowering external conditions, low morale, time pressures, fixed institutional attitudes and so on. There are no easy answers here, but therapists who seriously wish to use therapies that focus on developing and discovering new identities with their clients, need to reflect carefully upon their own identities first.

Developing identities through positive role models

One concrete way of demonstrating the expert role of people with aphasia is to offer employment that draws on their attributes, knowledge and skills. At the aphasia centre, people with personal experience of aphasia are employed in a variety of paid and unpaid roles, as counsellors, design experts for the production of promotional materials, teachers, workshop facilitators providing feedback to students and volunteers, actors and commentators in educational or awareness-raising videos, and even poets.

The skills and expertise of aphasic people can also be demonstrated, to themselves and others, by inviting their input to departmental or organisational procedures and membership of committees concerned with the running of the centre. Inevitably, this raises the problematic issue of tokenism. Time constraints, pressures on resources, and the need for sometimes painstaking negotiation and clarification of input can raise barriers to full involvement, no matter how good the intentions. These difficulties are not small or easily resolved. Another issue concerns payment, which can be problematic both from the point of view of the disabled person anxiously protecting his or her benefits, and from that of the budget-free therapist employer.

Making sense of aphasia

When one of our clients asked: 'Asphasia … dips … dispasia … what is asphasia?', he voiced a bewilderment which many people who come to the centre seem to experience. Understanding what aphasia is does not seem to come easily to anyone, including those who live with it themselves and those who witness its impact on friends and family members. Why is it that people with aphasia and those around them have such difficulty absorbing and digesting the many definitions and descriptions that doctors, therapists and other health workers helpfully provide over and over again, in written and spoken form? The difficulty seems to go far beyond any problems interpreting spoken and written language, although this is no small obstacle given the abstract and diverse nature of aphasia. Nevertheless, it seems certain that the process of learning to live with aphasia, resolving past experience and expectations for the future, and developing new, robust identities, has to start with an understanding and an acknowledgement of the nature of the changes which have occurred.

Clarifying the concept of aphasia

How good are therapists at explaining aphasia in a way that meaningfully captures the experience? Such a process demands a degree of creativity and sensitivity in developing aphasia-friendly representations. These have to make sense to those who have it and to their friends and family, and should accord with their experience. A flexibility of approach is useful, so that the therapist is ready to launch, say, into lengthy facilitated discussion or use drawings and videos and role-play to make the concept more clear.

As always, time can be an issue here. At the centre, we make frequent use of some excellent models of aphasia-friendly explanations of stroke and aphasia – for example, the booklet, *Drawing the Picture Together* which was published by the UK-based charity, Action for Dysphasic Adults (ADA). Another useful resource is the section on aphasia and competence in the *Pictographic Communication Resources Manual* (Kagan *et al*, 1996). We have also developed our own information resource, *The Aphasia Handbook*, which seeks to address aphasia and a range of other issues in an accessible format (Parr *et al*, 1999).

These materials can only benefit from the expansion, alteration and individualisation which come with shared discussion of personal experiences and interpretations. The therapeutic value of clarifying the concept of aphasia lies as much in the process of discussing and disentangling personal understandings as in the end product. The end product, however, which has developed its own form and authorship, will be 'owned' by the client and can be one way of establishing a point of reference for an otherwise intangible concept.

The visibility and comprehensibility of an impairment influences the process of adjusting to a different way of living and revising self and identity (French, 1994; Peters, 1996). For most people, aphasia is not visible, comprehensible or even consistent. These characteristics of aphasia offer a real challenge, both to the person struggling to make sense of the impairments, and to friends and relatives who often have neither the knowledge nor experience to shape their response to puzzlingly different communication.

Collaborative work with group members addressing these issues is described in the following sections of this chapter. In Chapter 4, group project work aimed at clarifying the concept of aphasia is also outlined.

To reveal or not to reveal?

French (1994) discusses the disclosure dilemmas faced by those whose impairment is invisible. Disclosure of aphasia is particularly perplexing. The choice to reveal that one has aphasia brings with it the risk of being thought stupid or incompetent, but the potential advantage of having one's needs for communicative support accommodated, at least to a degree. Conversely, concealing the aphasia might preserve others' perceptions of a competent adult while bringing the fearful disadvantage that the interlocutor will make no allowances for language impairment and breakdown in communication. This threat is consolidated by the additional fear of discovery and exclusion from 'normal' society. In the event, many people conceal aphasia by a variety of means including humour, feigning comprehension and avoiding active engagement in conversation.

Of course, the lack of public awareness about aphasia, the dearth of individuals who are skilled at supporting communication, together with the difficulties of actually undertaking such disclosure complicate the issue further. This may make concealment an entirely reasonable option. Not all people with aphasia will choose to disclose or feel comfortable revealing their communicative needs to others at all times.

However, people with different severities of aphasia have responded positively to the wallet-sized cards produced by the UK-based charities Action for Dysphasic Adults (ADA), the Stroke Association, and, more recently, as part of the *Aphasia Handbook* (Parr *et al*, 1999) which state that they have had a stroke and have a communication impairment. This is testimony to the value of supported disclosure. Effectively, these cards allow the person to identify, not only who they are and where they belong, but the nature of their impairment, and to place themselves as part of a community of people with aphasia. In other words, a card such as this can effectively affirm the personal and collective identities of people with aphasia.

Coping with ignorance

Inevitably, a person's concept of aphasia will be challenged, supported or misconstrued on an ongoing basis by others in daily life. Reactions and attitudes from family, friends, work colleagues, neighbours, service workers and strangers, many of whom may have little or no knowledge of aphasia, may serve to undermine, confuse or consolidate the person's concept of their communication impairment. Often the task of clarifying the nature and implications of aphasia falls to the very person for whom the ability to be clear and specific has been selectively damaged. The desire to educate and support others through the process of understanding aphasia, while grappling with the language impairment itself, can constitute an intensely frustrating experience.

Such frustrations are not aided by the rigidity of bureaucratic bandings of disability which have difficulty accommodating the complex, hidden nature of aphasia. Reflections on the difficulties faced by deaf people in constructing identities which are robust and inclusive of disability (Corker, 1998) could equally well apply to people with aphasia:

> As long as legislation attempts to squeeze sensory impairment into physical or mental categories there can be no comprehensive analysis of social, linguistic and attitudinal oppression. (Corker, 1998, p58)

Ignorance and lack of awareness as a barrier to accessing services and rights have been addressed in a number of places in this text. However, these issues are relevant to the development and maintenance of strong personal, social and collective identities.

Understanding aphasia: some therapeutic activities

Developing an aphasia-friendly leaflet

Translating complex written language into accessible, aphasia-friendly forms is not without linguistic, cognitive and creative demands. As a task, it is well suited to the 'more heads than one' approach which groupwork can offer. While the difficulty of not being able to please all people all of the time will be a feature of any group project, the agreements and disagreements of debate, and the understanding that springs from locating one's own concerns in relation to others, is often beneficial.

Having together determined a focus and audience for the leaflet (for example, an aphasia-friendly explanation of living with disability, or the translation of travel or benefits information for people with impaired reading skills), the first step will often be a clarification of what makes information accessible and inaccessible to people with aphasia. By reviewing various styles and formats for presenting information, using leaflets gathered from different sources, people with and without aphasia can identify and discuss preferences and levels of accessibility. Discussion (frequently summarised and clarified by the therapist) about vocabulary, grammar, size, type and amount of print, use of photographic material and layout will all form an important basis for future decisions about design and accessibility. An example is shown in Figure 5.1.

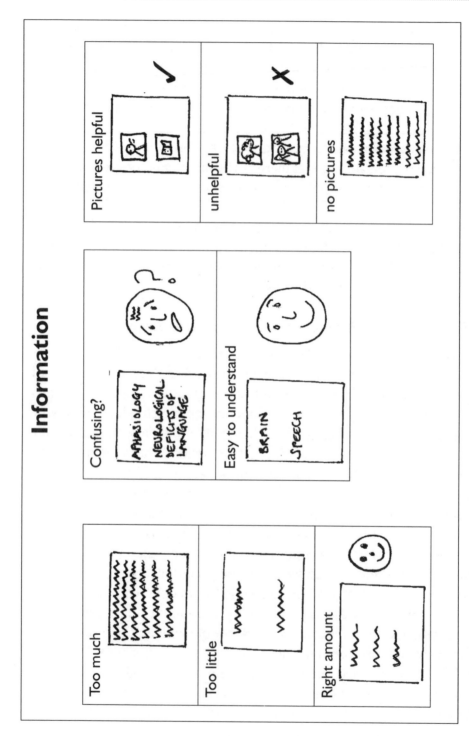

Figure 5.1 Developing accessible formats to represent information (1)

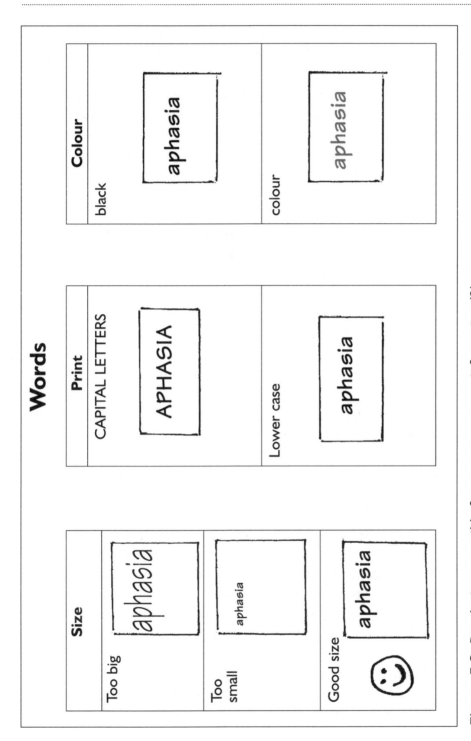

Figure 5.2 Developing accessible formats to represent information (2)

Such review activity is a means whereby people with aphasia can identify their particular needs and rights regarding the way information is presented. Multiple-choice formats, and systematic attention to wording, graphics and layout can offer useful market research opportunities with other people with aphasia. This promotes inclusion, participation and 'ownership' of the final product. Computer technology makes it easy to alter font size, style and spacing and to add graphics and icons. Generation of alternatives is quick and straightforward (*see* Figure 5.2).

The process of determining the topic will again require facilitated group discussion, design of alternatives and democratic, reasoned group decision. A common pitfall in this type of project work is the attempt to produce information which covers a multitude of issues not all of which will be equally relevant and pertinent to all members of the group. The group will benefit from constantly revisiting the aims and audience and restating rationales for decisions taken along the way. This can be done by a non-aphasic facilitator or a member of the group. Clarity, communication and assertiveness skills are essential to keep the team working towards a common goal. Within such negotiations there are many opportunities for group members to work towards more impairment-based therapy goals – for example, developing listening, summarising and clarifying skills.

The end product should be clear and accessible and may serve as an important resource for education of self and others. Many pieces of published information are too wordy, confusing and frequently unrelated to any disability which is not visible. The relief of making aphasia 'real' and tangible, and the intellectual and creative achievement of producing relevant and meaningful information (when the publicity departments of large public services and organisations have failed to do so, as evidenced in the forms and correspondence generated by social services and local council departments), provides substantial, positive proof of the competence and expertise of people with aphasia (*see* Figure 5.3).

Personalised definitions of aphasia

Leaflets or posters produced in a group context offer an overview of aphasia that enables individuals to locate themselves in relation to

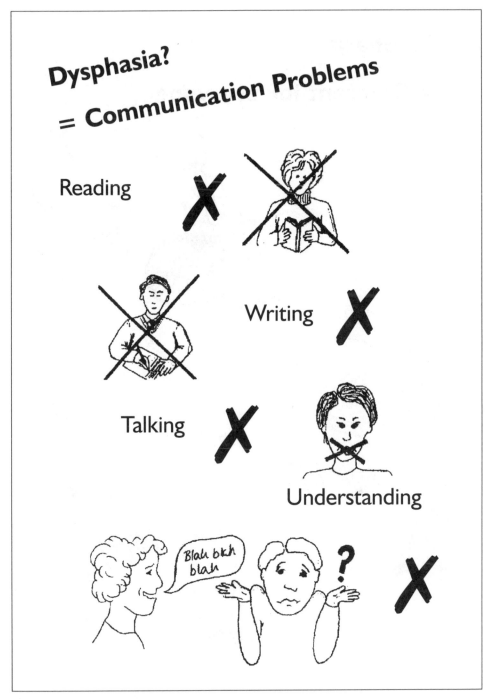

Figure 5.3 *What is dysphasia? – leaflet project*

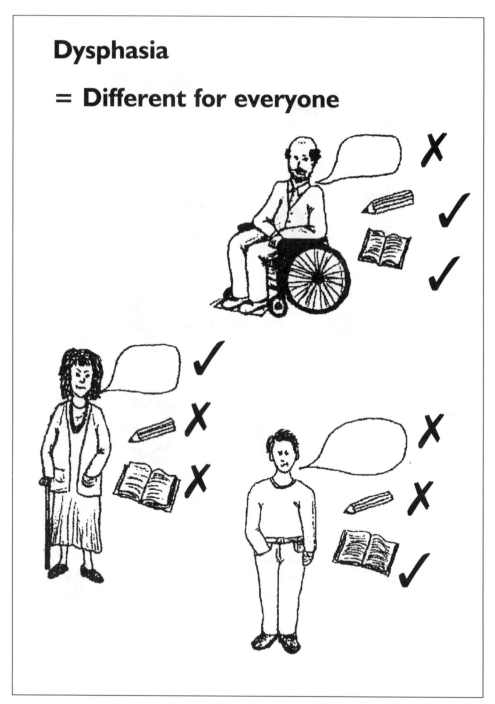

Figure 5.3 *Continued*

others, and to make sense of the breadth and complexity of aphasia. However, many people may also benefit from developing their own personalised definition of aphasia. Using the group definition or general published definitions as a starting point, individuals can highlight and graphically represent issues specific to their own aphasia.

This exercise could be carried out with a view to producing an all-purpose definition for use with family, friends and strangers, or for inclusion within a personalised communication file. For some, the activity may take on greater meaning if it is very specific – for example, personal guidelines for communicating with the doctor, a document informing an adult education tutor about communication needs, or an *aide-mémoire* for the person with aphasia and the solicitor engaged in decision making around personal finances. The nature of the interaction will therefore guide the amount of information and the specific details which might be included. A framework for developing personalised definitions of aphasia is shown in Table 5.1.

Table 5.1 *A framework for developing a personalised definition of aphasia*

Step	Resources/Supportive materials	Other issues
1 Identify possible areas of use for definition and statement of communication needs	• Knowledge of person's interests • Examples of previous difficulties communicating with those ignorant of aphasia	• Clarification of rationale • Relationship to other stated lifestyle goals
2 Review published definitions of aphasia and critically appraise for • content • style and personal preference of presentation	• ADA *Drawing the Picture Together* • PCRM (Kagan et al, 1996) • ADA *Medical Matters* video • Locally produced literature on aphasia • *The Aphasia Handbook* (Parr et al, 1999)	• Develop aphasia-friendly checklist/scales for critical appraisal

(continued)

Table 5.1 *continued*

Step	Resources/Supportive materials	Other issues
3 Elicit key headings relevant to own aphasia		• Be sure to include, if appropriate to the individual, headings beyond language, eg, time, fatigue, attitudes, competence
4 Develop a concise list of key statements/ graphic representations	• See, for example, Kagan *et al*, 1996 'What is Aphasia?'	• Remember to include strengths as well as impairments • Tick/cross icons can remind person (and conversation partner) of competencies as well as needs
5 Brainstorm communication needs/situations in selected environment	• For example, at the doctors, talking with family members, using the bus	
6 Discuss and note in relation to chosen situation: • way aphasic impairments impact on communication • way knowledge of this may help conversation partner		
7 Identify and list actions which conversation partner might take to make the interaction more enjoyable, easy, successful	• If necessary, derive actions from observation of role plays or conversation partnership videos where enabling/disabling actions of others are clearly apparent	• Use clear visual cues, eg, pictogram of person with aphasia and other clearly labelled to facilitate discussion of who in partnership is expected to do what
8 Clarify content so far in terms of • what is aphasia • how aphasia affects me • what you can do to help		

(continued)

Table 5.1 *continued*

Step	Resources/Supportive materials	Other issues
9 Negotiate format and presentation style	• Examples of presentation styles: +/– pictures • Listed information in different font sizes/styles (*see* Figs 5.1 and 5.2)	• Production could be carried out in further sessions together and could incorporate eg, impairment-based work on writing, self-monitoring of written output, keyword reading • Production of initial draft could also form project for volunteer, student, assistant, family
10 Review and amendment of produced draft for • content • format	• Use of checklists, as above	• Ensures person with aphasia has full participation in and control over decisions about definition while more time-consuming aspects of production may be completed by co-workers
11 Role-play of scenario/ situation which was identified in point 1. Video and review of • use of material • reactions of conversation partner • need for any further amendments	• Detail re potential use to craft role play as closely as possible to real-life situation • Observation checklist to guide video observation and evaluation of use of definition	

Making aphasia visible and comprehensible can support the process of adjustment, for the person with aphasia, their friends and family members. Group members have worked on producing:

1   A poster about the impact of aphasia.

2   Videos that explain what living with aphasia is like from the insider's perspective.

3   Videos that aim to demonstrate the communicative competence of people with varying degrees of aphasia.

4   Leaflets that describe for Members of Parliament the day-to-day reality of living with aphasia and how the benefits system fails to account for complex and often invisible welfare needs.

Such therapeutic ventures offer scope for self-exploration and personal development. Key issues of identity might be explored through discussion generated by the projects, which have to be sensitively facilitated. Topics which may arise in such discussions include:

- Attitudes and reactions to disability and aphasia
- Locating oneself now in relation to others, both with and without disability
- The abilities and expectations of people within the group in relation to past, present and future experiences

---

Case Study 5.1 Acknowledging aphasia: the cook's tale

Sheila was 61 when she had a left-hemisphere stroke leaving her with mild aphasia and a dense right hemiplegia. Prior to her stroke she worked in a number of creative, administrative roles, as a costume designer for a local theatre company, a charity administrator and a festival organiser. Her pastimes were also arts and entertainments based. Sheila lives with her husband and has two supportive adult children living locally.

Sheila came to the aphasia centre approximately one year after her stroke when outpatient therapy ceased. At this time, she had mild expressive language difficulties (some word-retrieval problems, spelling difficulty with longer, irregular words, function-word substitutions in writing, and mild/moderate difficulties reading longer length written material). However, Sheila's loss of confidence in all aspects of reading, writing and speaking was her most marked problem. Apart from her two weekly visits to a day centre, where she felt the other clients did not understand her communication difficulties or needs, opportunities to participate in everyday leisure activities were minimal.

Over a period of two years, Sheila received a package of individual and small group therapy, attending for one morning weekly to work on developing her confidence in her creative skills, learning to state her communication needs in a clear and assertive manner and exploring possible opportunities for accessing recreational activities. Sheila covered the following range of activities during this period:

- Developing a cookery book for one-handed cooks with aphasia-related reading difficulties
- Producing a video, entitled 'Living with Aphasia', to show other clients at the day centre
- Devising an aphasia-friendly map for people with aphasia who were visiting the centre for the first time
- Developing a personal definition of stroke and aphasia with a view to expressing her own physical and communicative needs to an adult education tutor

During these projects Sheila and her keyworker students had numerous opportunities to discuss her impairment and practise communication strategies (for example, highlighting key words to support reading, and discussing the nature of written and spoken words which would be predictably troublesome). It soon became obvious, however, that, if they were to help her develop confidence, those facilitating Sheila would need to shift the emphasis of therapy from language accuracy and focus instead on her sense of being a creative, competent producer and editor. Having previously used her communication skills to full effect in work and play, Sheila felt that she now lacked any powers of communication and had no skills to contribute to others. The rather ambitious project to develop a one-handed cookery book was a deliberate attempt to address this issue in a practical way, and to restore Sheila's faith in her own competence. This project therefore provides an interesting illustration of how shifting attention over time from Sheila's focus on language errors and inabilities to her creative potential and ability to 'write' a book can reinforce a person's confidence and sense of self. Significantly this new sense of self incorporates rather than seeks to deny or overcome the persisting reality of aphasia and disability. In Sheila's case, this situation led both to improvements in confidence levels and, importantly, to marked changes in her perception of her communication skills.

The cookery book project
Early negotiation of potential therapeutic goals associated with developing the cookery book sketched out a number of opportunities, some of which focused on the impairment. At the level of cognition and communication, for example, Sheila and her student keyworker were able to identify the following areas needing therapeutic attention:

- Refinement and practice of reading strategies for paragraph-length material
- Monitoring of accuracy in written output and identifying key areas (eg, correction of function-word substitutions)
- Organisation and planning to enable a manageable step-by-step approach to tasks
- Negotiating, setting and meeting deadlines
- Collaborative problem solving.

Development in each of these areas was built on an understanding both of the nature of the impairment and the way in which Sheila responded to it. Typically, she was quick to compare her current performance with her former competence, effectively undermining her confidence. Thus, it was important at this stage for her keyworker not only to listen to and acknowledge Sheila's expression of loss and frustration but also to model collaborative working. Sheila's impairments and their impact were not minimised in these interactions. However, they were approached from a perspective which emphasised skills and needs rather than one in which difficulties and imperfections were highlighted, tempting though it was for the student to work on the correct production of prepositions in sentence contexts.

Meanwhile the keyworker roles expanded to include conversation partner, scribe, monitor–evaluator, sounding board, confidence supporter and project team worker. Both partners developed in tandem the skills of negotiating, clarifying, delegating and clearly stating needs and anxieties. Themes of therapy relating more explicitly to the development of a stronger sense of personal and collective identity included the following:

1 *Personal identity*
- Raising awareness of personal strengths, skills and knowledge (for example, creativity, role in team, specific knowledge)
- Developing confidence in communication and life skills (for example, assertiveness, directing others)
- Raising awareness of needs, rights, the acceptability and means of accessing help (for example, use of therapist as a resource, use of word-processing facilities)
- Developing self-confidence and self-esteem in a project fed by high expectations and the hope of a tangible, high-quality end product

2 *Collective identity*
- Identification with other people with hemiplegia and reading impairment, particularly during the market research phase of the project
- Discussing needs and concerns shared by disabled people regarding restrictions on expectations and opportunities to participate

Sheila and her student keyworker also set themselves the task of identifying and dismantling barriers. In this context, the case was made that problems were imposed from without and that Sheila, as an individual, should not feel compelled to claim them as her own. Issues raised included:

- Circumventing physical barriers (for example, accessing information about tools for one-handed cooking)

- Identifying and problem solving language barriers (for example, critically appraising content, style, format of standard cookery texts). Sheila commented: 'The recipe books was quite ... mind-boggling, the printing and the layout and the ... too much waffle in them ...'
- Identifying and discussing financial barriers (for example, how loss of income can impact on a person's ability to afford more expensive ingredients)
- Identifying and discussing attitudinal barriers (for example, non-disabled people's assumptions regarding the cognitive and communication competence or recreational desires of people with disabilities)

Finally, some unexpected therapeutic opportunities arose with the interest excited by the project. Sheila's confidence grew with the positive feedback on the book which she received from visitors to the centre, friends and relatives. Similarly, other disabled people, therapists working in other rehabilitation settings and new student keyworkers were struck by her creativity and attention to detail. Through the role of educating and informing others, Sheila began to connect not only with a wide range of new acquaintances who viewed her as extremely able, but also with her communicative and competent pre-stroke self.

Evaluation

The cookery book project formed part of an integrated package of therapy. It is not easy to specify the changes arising from this component of therapy in isolation from the overall package of therapy. However, in an interview in which Sheila was asked about her perceptions of the project work, she highlighted changes in her confidence, communication abilities and sense of herself. Although these changes were captured on a variety of rating scales and measures of internal state used throughout her period of therapy, perhaps they are most clearly expressed in Sheila's own words:

'Oh God, it's just incredible really. Writing out the recipes and spelling and numeracy ... I never knew I was capable of writing a book and planning ... and designing it ... well sort of ... It's been remarkable really 'cos I've got so much pleasure and satisfaction and it's making me read and write better ... It's em ... confidence ... It's gradual and it's made me want to speak a lot more and communication with outsiders not just family.'

Sheila has sold a number of the completed recipe books containing 30 recipes (see Figure 5.4) and she is currently exploring ways of bringing the book to publication.

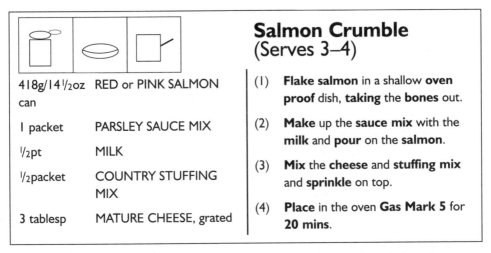

| 418g/14½oz | RED or PINK SALMON can | (1) | **Flake salmon** in a shallow **oven proof** dish, **taking** the **bones** out. |

Salmon Crumble
(Serves 3–4)

418g/14½oz	RED or PINK SALMON can
1 packet	PARSLEY SAUCE MIX
½pt	MILK
½packet	COUNTRY STUFFING MIX
3 tablesp	MATURE CHEESE, grated

(1) **Flake salmon** in a shallow **oven proof** dish, **taking** the **bones** out.

(2) **Make** up the **sauce mix** with the **milk** and **pour** on the **salmon**.

(3) **Mix** the **cheese** and **stuffing mix** and **sprinkle** on top.

(4) **Place** in the oven **Gas Mark 5** for **20 mins**.

Figure 5.4 *Example of an aphasia-friendly recipe for one-handed cookery*

Incorporating aphasia and disability into new lifestyles

Personal biographies and narratives

Within the fields of counselling, psychotherapy and sociology there is a long tradition of using patient narratives as a means of informing diagnosis and intervention, and as a means of understanding illness in the context of personal biography (Nettleton, 1995). More recently, 'narrative medicine' (pioneered by Kleinman, 1988 and Frank, 1995) has attracted the attention of mainstream medical practitioners including General Practitioners (Greenhalgh & Hurwitz,1999). Therapeutic approaches based on the process of listening and telling are to a certain extent compatible with social model principles, for a number of reasons.

1   Narratives allow for the affirmation of the client's expert role, as the 'voice of medicine' is separated from the 'voice of the lifeworld' (Mishler, 1984).

2   Involvement of the therapist as listener, questioner and supporter in the construction of the narrative allows the therapeutic relationship to be reconstrued. Instead of channelling an intervention, controlled by one party only and based on analysis of pathology, the relationship becomes a conversation in which the partners seek to understand, negotiate, clarify and chart new meanings and possibilities.

3   Through the value placed on the language, imagery and the story itself, the client's subjective experience of aphasia is affirmed rather than undermined.

It may be tempting for therapists to rush the person with aphasia into a restitution narrative. Frank (1995) warns against this and argues that a first step must be 'bearing witness' to the account given, which may be uncomfortably chaotic:

> Those living chaotic stories most certainly need help, but the immediate impulse of most would-be helpers is first to drag the teller out of this story, that dragging called some version of 'therapy'. Getting out of chaos is to be desired, but people can only be helped out when those who care are first willing to become witness to that story. Chaos is never transcended but must be accepted, before new lives can be built and new stories told. (Frank, 1995, p110)

The process of listening becomes a powerful foundation for diagnosis and intervention that is meaningful and acceptable to the ill or impaired individual, rather than generated by the objective, reductionist truths of science (Greenhalgh & Hurwitz, 1999). Narrative medicine has relevance for therapy, research and education. The challenge to the aphasia therapist comes in the form of learning to listen and being able to facilitate the telling. Often trained and experienced in counselling, many aphasia therapists will be aware of their own barriers to listening. Personal attitudes to disability, professional and organisational philosophies of intervention and constraints on time and resources are a few of the blocks that they face. Truly listening is no easy matter, as therapist researchers who have attempted to use in-depth interviewing can confirm. However, as some of the case studies reported later in this chapter reveal, it can be a powerful tool for driving both therapeutic interventions and the measurement of change. A reminder that 'for countless patients it is the telling of their story that helps to make them well' (Elwyn & Gwyn, 1999, p174), reaffirms the importance of supported conversation for individuals with aphasia and the creativity with which therapists might facilitate the telling in a practical, coherent way.

Portfolios and story telling

Many therapists working with adults with sudden acquired disability will have been struck by the starkness with which the pre- and post-illness identities are juxtaposed. We feel that this often difficult comparison can be directly addressed, rather than avoided, in therapy. Scrutinising pre- and post-illness photographs and discussions with the aphasic person, friends, family and colleagues are ways into the lived experience of aphasia. Such directness can introduce a new dimension and dynamic to therapy by acknowledging the past. This may be difficult in conventional rehabilitation, which, despite best intentions, is often geared to the present and the future.

Particularly in the acute stages of the impairment, the person with aphasia struggles to take in the new situation and may experience a profound sense of loss. The therapist's attempt to help the client adjust to his or her new reality and long-term prospect of living and coping with disability may be played out against a hazy, perhaps idealised, past and the uncertain reality of the present. The confusion is consolidated because language, the very means of clarifying what the situation is, is compromised. Personal portfolios can help to address powerful concerns in a structured, coherent way, and offer a record of the process and the outcome. The importance of such a tangible record seems to be related to the fact that, for people with compromised language, it can be difficult to tell the story of who they are and what happened. In addition, any gains in the struggle to understand may be lost if language is too fragile to hold them.

One of the primary therapeutic aims of personal portfolio work is the exploration, affirmation and concrete representation of a person's past and present as a means of moving more confidently and hopefully into the future. Unlike therapeutic approaches in which discussion of past lives and achievements is incidental, attention is focused on the person's biography and way of telling his or her life story. The idea of using portfolios with clients with aphasia developed from a small-scale research project investigating the meaning and benefits of self-advocacy groups for people with aphasia (Penman, 1998; Pound, 1998). We adapted work with people who have learning difficulties to the development of personal portfolios with individuals with aphasia and have subsequently used portfolios in both individual and group therapy sessions at the centre. Clients with more severe language impairments may choose to have their portfolios kept separately or integrated within communication books and files to highlight the links between identity, communication and self-expression (*see* Chapter 3).

What is a portfolio?

Personal portfolios may vary in form, style and content, but in general terms they can be described as:

- A collection of information about a person's past
- A source of information and examples about what is happening now
- A means of looking to the future through a statement of plans, ideas, goals and dreams.

The portfolio thus draws together aspects of a person's past, present and future, using a temporal sequence which characterises personal histories and narratives. The process of recalling, gathering, collating, selecting, explaining and representing biographical events and milestones forms the crux of the therapeutic experience and may address any or all of the following therapy themes:

- Building self-identity, self-esteem, self-value
- Seeing oneself in relation to others and checking out personal reality in relation to the perspective of others
- Exploring past and present relationships

- Identifying skills, strengths, limitations, needs
- Identifying barriers to well-being, whether external or self-imposed
- Identifying achievements and goals
- Representing and learning from experience
- Supporting the process of decision making
- Communicating about oneself with others as a way of self-exploration and personal development

In addition, the development of particular sections of the narratives can be easily integrated with impairment-based therapy goals, such as word-finding and vocabulary development, organisation of written language, divergent thinking and problem solving. Portfolio work has the potential to take the form of a fully coherent approach to disability which allows the person with aphasia to attempt to understand and 'improve' the impairment while learning to live with its persisting implications and consequences in a more comfortable way.

While an over-focus on the end product may interfere with the therapeutic potential already detailed, the concrete outcome of the personal portfolio can serve a range of functions which further support the development and re-negotiation of a post-illness identity. The person with aphasia can use the portfolio as:

- A tool to facilitate communication with others
- A lead-in to education and/or work
- A personal journal and method of self-analysis
- A record of gains and achievements

In addition, many people experience pride and confidence in creating something unique and personal (as with the cookery book project and creative writing). Stages in the development of personal portfolios are detailed in Table 5.2 and in Case Study 5.2.

The aims and activities detailed in this section by no means form a comprehensive list of the types of therapies that portfolio work can stimulate. Many of the specific examples are drawn from individual therapy sessions with a young woman with mild–moderate aphasia. Adaptations include greater use of pictorial material or writing support

Table 5.2 *Stages in the development of personal portfolios*

Aims of therapy (general)	Activity/Example	Useful resources/tips
I Demonstrate potential and underlying rationale of portfolio work	• Show client examples of portfolios • Highlight changes/ therapeutic benefits for those clients whose portfolios are used	• Collect samples of portfolio work from other clients, illustrating range of people, impairments, presentation and style preferences
2 Identify impairment and non-impairment based goals of therapy which portfolio work may address	• Goal setting based on listening and personal relevance	• See Chapter 2 on goal setting
3 Identify framework and timescale for portfolio work Prioritisation of therapy aims	• Brainstorm possible headings/sections for portfolio, eg, family, work, interests, stroke, rehabilitation, achievements, dreams • Select starting point, possible content and relationship of work on this section with specific therapy aims	• Examples of other portfolios • Therapist develops own personal portfolio as way of considering content/ selection issues • Typed list of potential therapy aims from (2) to cross reference to section content
4 Clarify roles of therapist/ client in constructing portfolio Develop client's confidence in personal skills and autonomy	• Brainstorm materials, resources, skills required to compile first section • Identify personal expertise and needs from others • Allocate tasks, roles in collection, selection, presentation of material	• Portfolio examples to show use of photos, computer technology, handwriting, drawings • Examples of alternative design and layout

(continued)

Table 5.2 *Continued*

Aims of therapy (specific)	Activity/Example	Useful resources/tips
5 To identify personal attributes and achievements	• Using timelines or illustrated decades, select highlights relating to work, home, interests • Relate these key events to a personal attribute • Ask a significant person to write a testimonial/ personal letter of commendation about you	• Use photographs and known autobiographical information to support elicitation • Use experiences, suggestions of other group members to probe areas of achievement • Feedback of group/ therapist to relate past achievements to current reality
6 To identify and acknowledge progress	• Identify milestones in recovery • Identify points of change in communication, mobility, confidence • Draw/write 3 significant experiences/words from: a) time of stroke; b) 6 months after; c) now	• Narratives relating to hospital and rehabilitation experiences • Choose representative blobby person or card/ art images to represent and discuss different points in distant and recent past and present
7 To develop confidence in using coping strategies	• Select a situation/activity which you previously avoided or were unable to do • Describe how you approach the problem now • Develop a list of tips for yourself/others who find themselves in similar tricky situations	• Aphasia-friendly questionnaires to elicit stressful/difficult situations • Comparison of daily activities at time of stroke, return home, now

(continued)

207

Table 5.2 Continued

Aims of therapy (specific)	Activity/Example	Useful resources/tips
8 To identify and participate in social networks To locate self and strengths/limitations in relation to others	• Represent significant people, friends, helpers a) at time of stroke/illness b) in rehabilitation phase c) in current phase of recovery • Use dotted and heavy lines to indicate strength/power of relationship • Identify potential additions to social network in future	• Use of drawing, multiple-choice names, buttons/stones to represent people • Use of colour, spatial organisation, in relation to central figure of client to differentiate types and strength of relationships • Discussion and probing to elucidate roles, contributions and motivations of individuals within the network
9 To identify future ambitions and directions To clarify and explore new opportunities relating to education/work/leisure To identify needs relating to any future activities	• Write a curriculum vitae of past and current strengths, skills and achievements • Identify previously unidentified personal resources and self-growth resulting from experience of disability • Identify successfully negotiated challenges of living with disability • Match personal skills and interests with potential work/recreational opportunities in local area	• See next section of chapter re developing CV • Use of cue cards with personal attributes/skills for group members to allocate to others in the group
10 To develop effective use of writing strategies (eg, dictionary, thesaurus, word-processing functions) to support written expression	• Critical analysis of baseline written description • Elaboration of passage using expanded vocabulary • Practical activities using computer thesaurus, spell check, etc.	• Relate to assessments of written language production • Negotiate agreed level of accuracy • Comparison (? and inclusion) of before/after examples in portfolio to represent and demonstrate change

from the therapist or support worker – for example, in the form of captions for photographs. Pictographic representations of past and present life (as described by Kagan *et al*, 1996) are also possible.

Case Study 5.2 Telling the story: the Personal Portfolio Group
The Personal Portfolio Group met together for 15 once-weekly afternoon sessions, lasting between 60 and 90 minutes. Many of the therapy themes related to those in other ongoing individual and group sessions that participants were attending (for example, conversation skills, poetry and aphasia, and project work).

The group consisted of seven people with mild–moderate aphasia, aged between 43 and 64 years. Time post-onset of aphasia varied between 18 months and 3 years. The group was facilitated predominantly by two speech and language therapy students, with help from a supervising clinician. The group was largely exploratory, but its primary aims were to:

• Increase understanding of aphasia in the context of personal biography
• Identify and represent personal strengths, skills and achievements
• Explore personal goals for the future and facilitate change in social interaction and participation
• Provide opportunities to practise and generalise individual communication and life skills

Sessions typically followed a two-pronged approach: discussing issues of identity and working on the task of developing portfolios. Group members' preferences as to content, organisation and style of the portfolios varied considerably, as did skills and speed of decision making, writing and presentation. Juggling individual preferences, skills and aims with a group focus and agenda was not always easy. Some group members, for example, were dependent on a considerable amount of support to write up or present sections, while other members were happy, once having decided on a section, to go off and complete this independently at home. Some people were skilled at word processing while others had little notion of the ways this might

---

209

support presentation. Some members could easily list achievements from their past and present, while others needed considerable support to identify positive aspects of themselves before and, more particularly, after their stroke. Some members would routinely bring in supporting material from home (such as photographs and certificates) while others rarely brought such memorabilia.

However, the diversity of group members' experience, style and ability could also work positively in the sharing and affirming of personal experiences and individual skills. A member of the group who was initially reluctant to work on his own portfolio, because, as he said, 'I can't do any of the jobs me did before', was persuaded to use his computer skills to scan in pictures and copy words. He produced beautiful colour prints of other group members' words and images. By the time the project came to an end, he had produced his own graphic portfolio containing scenes and stories from his pre-stroke life together with more recent achievements relating to his representations of brain damage and life within the group.

Feedback from others in activities focusing on self-presentation and self-characterisation was also beneficial. Using pictures, keywords and cards describing aspects of personality, individuals within the group identified key self-perceptions relating to the pre- and post-aphasia self. The rest of the group then acted as an objective witness to these statements, thereby providing the basis for reality testing and comparison of internal perceptions and external views. Thus one person who carried with her a strong feeling of intellectual inferiority (partly springing from her own negative perceptions of disabled people and partly because she had been forced to abandon her PhD studies) had this view firmly contradicted by the group's strong identification of her as an intellectual and a thinker.

Some of the tasks that were undertaken by the Portfolio Group are presented below. Some group members chose to retain the definitions and lists produced in sessions as an explicit part of their portfolio. Others preferred a more individually determined style of presentation and kept these materials separate. Nevertheless, key themes of looking at past, present and future and the perceptions and illustrations of self became part of the infrastructure of the portfolios.

Portfolio activities

1 Who am I?

Group members list key attributes which they feel mark them as individuals. For example:

I ... am Isobelle Marie

I ... am independent

I ... love red wine

I ... have a degree in politics

2 Testimonials

Assign cards describing personality traits to different individuals in the group. Develop a testimonial based on this selection of words together with other thoughts on the individual's personal attributes and qualities. This activity could be supported by asking a friend or colleague to write a personal reference. Testimonials should be honest and clear with a focus on the points and characteristics which really define and make the individual valued and unique. They should be written in the present tense and make reference to recent as well as past events, thus providing opportunities to integrate the person's pre- and post-stroke self.

3 Representing past, present and future

Using a range of postcards, greeting cards and art images, ask individuals to select an image which represents their thoughts and feelings:

- At the time of their stroke/illness
- As they feel about themselves now
- As they might like to be in the future

This activity, recorded and discussed, can provide a window on personal identity, offer a structured opportunity to develop narratives relating to new biography and elicit feedback from others regarding the personal journey.

4 Highlights and lowpoints

Developing lists relating to positive and negative aspects of certain areas of experience can be a further way of facilitating narratives and gaining perspective on traumatic events. This can also give a solid and practical framework for accessing experiences which might otherwise remain concealed. Furthermore, by placing a numerical limit on choices, group participants are encouraged to be relatively concise in representing themselves to others. This can both pre-empt overlong and egocentric elaborations on self and also distil a person's unique characteristics, providing a clear pathway through what could be a linguistic and experiential maze.

Examples of highlight and lowpoint lists might include:

- The *five* best and worst things about childhood
- The *five* most significant people in your life
- The *five* best and worst things that happened to you in hospital
- People who have been most (and least) supportive since you had your stroke
- *Five* milestones in your recovery.

Conversation about these issues can be usefully supported with photographs, time lines, pictographic or written cue cards and worked examples. The process of representing these issues verbally and visually within a person's portfolio can give individuals both permission and a practical way of discussing important memories and experiences with peers, therapists, facilitators, family and friends.

5 Personal statements of strengths, skills and needs

Many people with aphasia have a strong sense of skills, networks and lifestyle options which have been negatively affected by the onset of communication and physical disability. They are often less explicit about skills, strengths, talents and qualities which living with a disability can reveal. These can include resourcefulness, compassion, ability to listen, clarity and directness of expression, as well as the range of human skills and qualities that individuals have developed in their home, leisure and work life. Listing and eliciting strengths and qualities from others can be a way of beginning to redress the balance.

A second stage involves being clear and explicit in stating the limitations that aphasia has imposed and the related actions that people in the external environment may take to accommodate or circumvent these difficulties. Thus, if someone has an auditory processing impairment, a conversation partner may be required to do the following:

- Treat the person with aphasia as a competent adult
- Repeat or slow down spoken information
- Write down keywords
- Allocate time to communicate in an unhurried, relaxed way

The curriculum vitae

Many people who come to the centre have the experience of applying for jobs and courses and of trying to sell their strengths to potential employers, tutors and others. A similar disclosure of identity and personality occurs early on in friendships and relationships. The preparation or revision of a curriculum vitae (CV) is often helpful in these processes, and can form a useful basis for people with acquired disability in reaffirming their past and looking to the future.

Devising or revising a CV offers the opportunity to revisit former activities, interests and achievements. Of course, this can be an emotional experience for people whose newly acquired communication and physical impairments mean those experiences and activities are no longer possible. However, acknowledging these losses, within a context of admiration and interest for the pre-stroke identity and integration with the person now, can be a powerful and concrete way of connecting past and present concepts of self. The nature of a CV also allows people with aphasia to contemplate and articulate their hopes for the future in an assertive way.

Again, this identity-focused activity works well within a supportive group context. Group members can work together to extract, identify and feed back on each other's past skills and future potential – attributes which individuals may well lose sight of. The facilitator provides frameworks and practical conversational support for the telling of past experiences and the extracting of personal abilities. Regular clarification, restatement and summary is another language-based skill which the facilitator can offer, both to the group and to individuals. This keeps the range of personal, educational, recreational and work attributes firmly in view.

Caregiving: negotiating new identities

Just as suddenly acquired impairment catapults the individual with aphasia into a new phase of personal biography and re-evaluation of identity, so too caregivers of people with aphasia experience profound changes to their own personal and social identity. One of the caregivers who attended a support group for relatives at the centre remarked: 'I know that his life has changed but mine has as well. I've lost my freedom.' (Pound & Parr, 1998) In a qualitative evaluation of the group, in which they took part in in-depth interviews, caregivers identified the wide-ranging impact of their partners' aphasia upon their own identity and lifestyle. They highlighted, among other things, changes in social and family networks, feelings of inadequacy in managing the 'caring role', and their loss of agency and control vis-à-vis the present and future.

The caregivers offered narratives that were rich with examples of stress, chaos, uncertainty and isolation. They expressed the sense of submergence and loss of self within the new caregiving role, particularly when they had to give up their own career in order to devote time to the person with aphasia. Caregivers struggled to bear the strain of being with and supporting their partners at all times and to cope with persistent fatigue. They also had to deal with external difficulties, battling to claim services, entitlements and benefits, access relevant and comprehensible information and handle the responses and attitudes of friends, family and strangers to the changes in their lives.

Rice *et al* (1987) summarise the benefits that support groups for relatives can offer in terms of information, psychological support and improved functional communication. Techniques for working with relatives to enhance conversation support skills and collaborative systems of interaction and transaction are described in Chapter 3. In this chapter, we address therapies which facilitate caregivers in the appraisal and re-construction of their own identity, following the onset of aphasia.

Warm-up activities

Many caregivers, particularly when the aphasia and other impairments are severe, rapidly become caught up in the illness, rehabilitation schedules and day-to-day requirements of the disabled person. It is often the case that, when asked to tell the group about themselves, caregivers focus entirely upon the disabled person, their illness, their losses, their needs, talking about themselves only incidentally and in relation to this point of reference. For this reason, warm-up activities that draw out and reinforce the identity of the caregiver, his or her strengths, skills and personalities, can be useful starting points. The focus of such warm-up activities falls upon encouraging the caregiver to talk about him- or herself as an individual with a past, present and future, not merely as a caregiving appendage.

To this end, participants might be invited to state one past achievement, one secret from their past and one hero or heroine they might like to meet. An alternative approach might be for participants to select decades and relate a personal story associated with that period in their life. They can also be asked to draw a timeline representing birth to the present and to identify five highlights in the form of events which have happened to them during their lifetime. In each case, the aim is to focus the caregiver on his or her own life and biography, reinforced by the attention of the group, rather than upon the needs of his or her disabled partner.

'Public' and 'private' narratives

Many caregivers stress the isolation of their situation and the feeling of being compelled to play a role for which they are often both untrained and unprepared. Within our culture, there are high expectations of the caregiving role: caregivers are expected, among other things, to be tolerant, uncomplaining, dedicated and self-sacrificing. Social accounts of the devoted caregiver leave little room for emotions such as anger, resentment, guilt and feelings of anxiety and uncertainty in the day-to-day process of living with illness and disability. Unsurprisingly, these emotions feature prominently in caregivers' narratives. Thus, the 'public' narrative of caregiving is often at odds with the 'private' narrative.

Facilitated discussions which allow these powerful emotions to come to the surface and which directly address their lack of acceptability can be a first step to validating the caregiver as an individual. Stories and examples of difficult or successful negotiation of an everyday situation (perhaps relating to communication, going out or visiting others) can be shared by the group. This scenario then becomes an important test ground for ideas and a source of feedback. Listening to similar and diverse experiences of others in caregiving situations and contributing his or her own experience, the caregiver can tap into a powerful source of new ideas and experience a surge of confidence from the affirmation of others. Telling one's story and being listened to by a supportive and empathetic audience can be critical in the revision and reappraisal of personal and collective identity.

It is useful if the sharing of experience can be captured in a tangible and practical form and this can be done by generating lists of tips and guidelines for participants to take away. The participants can gather strategies relating to a range of issues – for example, managing anger or guilt, or making mobility restrictions easier to live with. Developing these lists with real-life examples and the actual wording used by individuals in the group further validates personal experience, connects isolated people with each other and can lead to a growth in confidence and a sense of making a real contribution.

Developing new perspectives

In their evaluation of support groups at the aphasia centre, participants identified one of the positive outcomes as a newfound ability to integrate caregiving into life as a whole, rather than being overtaken and engulfed by it. They attributed this change to the sharing of experiences, the ability to take time out and reflect on the process of caregiving in the company of others, and the development of new practical coping strategies such as being more assertive and feeling less guilty about requesting help from others. Participants also valued practical activities around recognising and prioritising their own needs, and goal setting.

One method of putting caregiving firmly into context and re-establishing perspective has been borrowed from a self-help manual which tackles fear and lack of confidence (Jeffers, 1987). Constructing a 'lifestyle grid' (*see* Figure 5.5) enables people to identify the range of important components of their life and the time they allocate to each aspect. Many

Sandra's Lifestyle Grid

Before stroke

Family Seeing sisters	Work	Work
Work	Family Seeing grandchildren	Home Decorating Maintenance
Hobbies – dancing club	Time with Sam	Relaxing at home

After stroke

Hospital/day centre + Sam	Shopping Housework	Appointments Travel + Sam
Home with Sam	Home with Sam	Home with Sam
Home with Sam	Home with Sam	Family

Figure 5.5 *Sandra's lifestyle grids*

people who come to the centre find that the lifestyle grids help them to identify in a concrete and visual way the disproportionate amount of time they spend with, caring for or worrying about the disabled person.

Discussion of the lifestyle grids, perhaps with reference to pre-stroke/injury patterns, is a useful, concrete way of acknowledging the major changes brought by the caregiving role. Clearly, a radical overhaul of lifestyle will not be a realistic option for most people. However, it is possible to use the grids as a basis for setting realistic goals, and perhaps implementing change in one small component of the overall pattern. An example of this process is given in Table 5.3. Sandra became a full-time caregiver at the age of 51, when her husband had a severe stroke which

Table 5.3 *Goal setting for change – Sandra*

Stage/Aim of therapy	Activity	Resulting issues/ Clinical reflections
1 Identify current overview of lifestyle	Complete lifestyle grid	• Virtually all areas relate to husband's needs • No time prioritised for self
2 Identify barriers to change	Discussion of why Sandra has no time for self	Emergence of feelings of guilt, anxiety that husband will fall or have fit if left, need to promote 'coping' front to 'protect' children
3 Identify one area of change, one activity she would like to pursue	Discussion of previous lifestyle, what activities she misses	• Sandra spoke of her love of socialising and dancing • Now impossible due to (a) anticipated guilt of enjoying herself, (b) fear of leaving husband, (c) inability to ask others for help
4 Set realistic goal, relating to an opportunity to go dancing	Goal-setting process: • worked example using group facilitator/other group members • defining and refining a goal that is Specific, Measurable, Achievable, Realistic and Time bound (SMART)	Goal determined as 'Sandra will go dancing once with her sisters before the follow-up group in six weeks' time'

Table 5.3 *Goal-setting for change – Sandra*

Stage/Aim of therapy	Activity	Resulting issues/ Clinical reflections
5 Identify necessary steps, people, resources required to enable outing	• Revisit barriers to going out • Set sub-goals for each of these identifying timescale and practical/people resources required – for example, (a) by x date Sandra will contact daughter to discuss plan (b) by x date Sandra will ring sisters to ask them to organise night out	• Discussion of guilt and group reinforcement of right and importance of occasional prioritisation of own life and needs to cope in longer term • Discussion of barriers – real and imagined – to accessing support from other family members • Problem solving and scripting re approaches to asking daughter to stay with husband while Sandra out
6 Emotional and verbal preparation for planning	• Visualising discussion of event with husband, sisters, daughter to anticipate and prepare for own and others' reactions • If necessary, problem solving and role play	Group members listen to but also challenge and suggest alternative possible scenarios for proposed interactions: eg, husband and others may get pleasure from seeing her enjoying self; other family members may be keen to help but don't know how
7 Review of event and whether goal achieved	Discussion of goals achieved/ changed and problems arising in follow-up group	Sandra had gone dancing twice since previous group. She reported her enjoyment of both events and the unanticipated ease of enlisting support. Her husband had been delighted at how smart and happy she looked and her daughter had recounted how pleased she and the other children were that she was looking after herself

left him with mobility impairments and marked aphasia. Eighteen months after his stroke, she joined the support group at the centre.

Participation and aphasia

Living in the 'borderlands': isolation and marginalisation

The negative cycle of reduced participation, restricted access to conversation and diminished connection to the everyday life of the community has been well documented. Holland & Beeson (1993), Kagan (1995), Lyon et al (1997), Simmons-Mackie (1998) and Byng et al (1999) describe the challenges faced by the aphasia therapist in facilitating access and reconnection. The onset of aphasia and other acquired impairments will frequently affect an individual's ability to participate in the transactions and interactions underpinning most relationships, and work and leisure activities. Faced with the sudden loss or change of established personal, social, familial and work identities, many people are understandably bewildered to find themselves acquiring a new identity. Suddenly, they become 'disabled', and are expected to adapt to a label which will have many personal and social connotations, not always positive.

It would be easy at this point to individualise the experience of aphasia in terms of a personal loss and a valiant battle to cope with the impaired body and compromised communication. Understandably, many people with acquired disabilities struggle to be as 'normal' as possible and the desire to be restored may be ongoing. The individual's personal story may have changed dramatically, but in the external communication environment the rules and expectations around social interaction are powerfully maintained. The person with impaired communication can no longer adhere to those rules, and therefore enters into a marginalised state. Many people describe the growing sense of being excluded, different, 'other'. The dissonance between individual perceptions and the responses of others can lead to a sense of bewilderment and dislocation as the disabled individual attempts to construct new private narratives which incorporate the experience of impairment.

Thomas (1999), Hogan (1999) and, famously, Sontag (1978) use territorial and citizenship metaphors to express their personal struggles to locate themselves in the experience of illness and disability. They inhabit the area between disabled and non-disabled worlds: *the 'borderlands'*. They struggle for connectedness. One way to reconnect is to get rid of the impairment, or conceal it, or become locked in a struggle to eradicate it. Another way is through meeting, relaxing, interacting and campaigning with other disabled people, developing new social connectedness, in ways which challenge representations of impairment as shameful, unsightly and bad. It is not easy to develop and sustain self-value and confidence as a disabled person. Writing about her own impairment, Thomas (1999) says:

> The long history of hiding my impairment has meant that it is second nature to me now. There is thus a disjuncture between my sense of 'who I am' (a disabled woman) and the sense of 'who she is' held by most other people who know me. This means that much of the time I am in the 'borderlands' between the disabled and non-disabled worlds, and I suspect that this is a very common experience for people like me who have impairments which, for one reason or another, are not obvious (Thomas, 1999, pp54-55).

The activities described in this section are an attempt to enable people with aphasia to explore and develop new narratives of impairment. Challenging the predominant discourses which represent impairment as incompetence, they offer one way of enabling people with aphasia to develop a sense of their own power and value.

Identifying barriers to participation

Many therapists will be aware how readily aphasic individuals claim responsibility for breakdowns in communication. They have the communication impairment; therefore they take the blame for problems. The aphasia (and the person who has it) are deemed responsible for access to friendships, work, leisure activities and participation in life becoming restricted. Many individuals with recently acquired impairments have little experience of living within a disabled world but long-established ideas (reinforced by stereotypes in literature, drama, advertising and the media) of disabled people as victims of misfortune, figures of pity, evil or bizarre misfits. It is hardly surprising that problems disabled people face are seen in terms of the natural consequences of an individual's impairment, rather than the oppressive, disabling barriers erected by an able-bodied society.

Activities which make explicit and seek to challenge these disabling barriers are discussed more fully in Chapter 4. However, they re-emerge here as an important step towards the reconstruction of public, social and cultural narratives of disability. The approach described in this text draws the attention of the person with aphasia to alternative models of disability, the problems imposed by a disablist society, and creative approaches to informing and educating others about their competence, rights and needs.

Self-help, self-advocacy and other models of group support

In the UK, the charity Action for Dysphasic Adults (ADA) has done much to support the growth of self-help groups among the community of people with long-term aphasia. Offering practical help in the form of workshops, manuals and advice from development staff, ADA has worked collaboratively to support people with aphasia who wish to meet together regularly and to develop their own group agenda. Membership of this national network of groups brings numerous diverse benefits to people with aphasia (Coles & Eales, 1999).

Self-help groups, like other groups of people with a shared disability, provide participants with the opportunity to locate themselves within a new and alternative world. In this, they enjoy the security of a group of people who have also endured the prejudices and unaccommodating practices of the non-disabled world. Inevitably, the practice of self-help varies. Some groups take a directly political approach to the situation in which they find themselves, actively campaigning and awareness raising. Some are content to maintain close links with a supporting speech and language therapy organisation, while others may prefer to seek new alliances within the field of disability organisations. Some groups struggle to find a guiding philosophy and coherent identity as different members place different emphases on the social, political and therapeutic activities. No matter how the group identity develops or how long members continue to meet, the opportunities which such groups provide for telling personal stories and hearing the experiences of others are generally highly valued.

Supporting self-help groups: the role of the therapist
The role of the speech and language therapist in working with and supporting the setting up and development of self-help groups is not always easy. Dilemmas for the therapist concern finding funding for time to support the group as it sets up, when and how to withdraw, how to allocate time and non-directive support as the group continues and how to assist the group to manage the numerous problems which are likely to arise. Typical problems concern the recruitment of new members, the management of over-dominant group members, and clarifying the distinction between speech and language therapy and self-help. The UK-based charity, Action for Dysphasic Adults (ADA) can offer help and advice for groups in the UK, but some of the following questions may support therapists in being clear about their liaison role in relation to the self-help group.

- What do you/potential group members understand by empowerment?
- What is your motivation/your organisation's motivation for supporting the development of a self-help group?
- What values, style/model of management might best support a self-help ethos?
- How does self-help differ from therapist- or volunteer-led groups?
- Consider your personal approach to and experience of power sharing with clients.
- What would you consider acceptable/unacceptable for a self-help group to do?
- What skills and attitudes would you consider appropriate in aphasic/therapist leaders of a self-help project?

In addition, the following questions relating to *practical issues* should be addressed.

- How much time can you allocate to the project?

- What are the funding requirements: (a) to support you in setting up the group; (b) to support the group on an ongoing basis (for example, accommodation costs)?
- Who will you identify as practical sources of support: (a) among your managers; (b) among colleagues; (c) among aphasic clients?
- What timescale will the setting-up period cover?
- How will you recruit members?
- How will you support aphasic people in negotiating (and regularly reaffirming/re-negotiating) management issues (for example, setting up ground rules, determining philosophy of the group, accessing a meeting place)?
- How will you support aphasic members in developing communication skills which enable the inclusion of people with different levels of aphasia in the group?
- What level and type of input does the group want/can the group expect from you/the therapy service?
- How will you facilitate networking between this group and other relevant groups/organisations?
- How can you ensure the group is aware of the range of potential directions/activities which they might pursue (for example, can visits be arranged to other established groups)?
- What will the procedure be for ongoing liaison with you and your organisation?

Other models of group support which promote collective identity

Self-help is not the only form of groupwork which may facilitate the development of confidence and growth through the exploration of collective identity. We have used other models of groupwork to explore particular identity themes. These include:

1   *Women's Group.* This focuses on issues around parenting, sexuality, work, further education and assertiveness.
2   *Young Persons' Group.* This focuses on attitudes and perceptions of the public regarding young people with disabilities, access to work, benefits and rights, developing and maintaining relationships.

3   *Relatives' Group.* This addresses issues around caregiver identities, both new and old.

4   *'Living with Aphasia' Group.* This identifies issues which people face in their everyday life – for example, coping with ignorance and stigma, dealing with the health service and accessing information.

5   *Conversation Group.* Group members explore views and opinions on topics in the news, through social conversation in a relaxed, unhurried environment. Although this is not always easily accomplished, group members aim to develop awareness of conversational support needs in order to ensure the inclusion and participation of people with more severe aphasia. (The dilemmas which arise are detailed in Chapter 3.)

6   *Self-Advocacy Group.* This is an alternative form of self-help in which discussion and activity are more explicitly political.

The main challenge facing these groups arises in balancing cohesion and focus with the diversity brought by individual members. However, the dynamic relationship between the individual and group is often very positive, enabling participants to 'find their bearings' with reference to the experience and opinions of others. Case Study 5.3 is an example of how a focus on personal and public issues in aphasia can promote a sense of location and self-worth.

Case Study 5.3 The Self-Advocacy Group

The Self-Advocacy Group was one of two experimental groups which ran over a 10-week period with a view to evaluating the potential relevance, needs and benefits of a self-advocacy model to people with aphasia. The work was supported by the Ajahma Trust and has been reported elsewhere by Penman (1998).

Eight participants were recruited through local therapists and from therapy groups at the aphasia centre. All had expressed an interest in exploring issues of confidence, lifestyle and speaking out for themselves as people with aphasia. Participants varied in age (43–67 years), time post-onset (2–10 years) and severity of aphasia. Given the short timescale of the group, people with severe receptive aphasia or people who were likely to require considerable support in the group environment were excluded.

The group met for two hours weekly. It was co-facilitated by a speech and language therapist and a person with teaching and groupwork skills, as well as aphasia. This partnership offered a practical model of power sharing and an opportunity for the therapist to develop and monitor a non-directive role within the group. The agenda of the group was decided in pre-course interviews and opening discussions.

The content of the course was loosely pre-determined by the facilitators and an advisory panel comprising three people with personal experience of stroke and aphasia. However, it largely took a flexible approach to discussion and problem solving as guided by the participants. Over 10 weeks, the following topics were covered:

1 *Personal experience*
- Biographies: telling personal stories about life before, during and after the onset of aphasia
- Portfolio work: developing a personal portfolio (see earlier in this chapter) to represent life experience as a non-disabled and disabled person

2 *Attitudes and approaches to aphasia and disability*
- Models of disability; living with disability
- Internal/external barriers: identifying barriers imposed by self or others
- Discrimination faced as a person with aphasia and other impairments

3 *Practical problems and coping strategies*
- Dealing with anger, anxiety, guilt
- Personal relationships.
- Dealing with doctors, welfare agencies and structural barriers to accessing support
- Coping with time pressure
- Developing confidence and assertiveness techniques as a person with aphasia

- Educating others about the strengths, difficulties and needs of people with aphasia

4 *Conversations and repair*
  - Identifying options/preferences/responsibilities of the aphasic and non-aphasic person in conversation
  - Identifying the skills and characteristics of good and bad conversation partners

The discussions arising within these topics were wide-ranging and included:

- The meaning of advocacy and self-advocacy
- Implications of living with a disability and ageing with a disability
- Expectations of recovery, past and present
- The hidden nature of aphasia; dealing with its intangibility
- The possible impact of the recently passed Disability Discrimination Act
- Attitudes towards claiming benefits
- Using illness and aphasia as a scapegoat for pre-existing relationship problems
- The effect of retirement on communication and relationships
- How caregivers cope with role change
- Training for caregivers
- The impact of aphasia and disability on children
- Coping with guilt, fear, vulnerability and dependency
- Making information accessible
- Finding paid employment.

As can be seen from this list of topics, the group focused on issues around living with a disability. Communication and communication change were addressed, but only within this context. Issues were explored through supported conversation and discussion and through more structured, activity-based work on portfolios, barriers and strategies. Each group member set personal goals related to advocacy, and some of these were addressed within session time. For example, one participant wanted to role-play assertiveness techniques for making her mother wait and listen to her opinion. Another participant set a goal around managing her anger when communicating with her daughter.

The therapist-facilitator was charged with summarising and writing up the minutes of each meeting. Sessions were also video recorded to support members who were absent and to use as a record and means of clarifying points previously discussed. Both facilitators checked at regular intervals with group members that the style of facilitation and manner of supporting conversation were appropriate.

Evaluation

The group was evaluated via an eclectic package of measures including:

- Pre- and post-course in-depth interview undertaken and analysed by independent researchers
- Aphasia-friendly scales of internal state
- Shortened Ryff Psychological Well-Being questionnaire (Thelander *et al*, 1994)
- Audit of individual goal attainment
- Completion of personal portfolio

The changes noted by group participants can be summarised as follows:

1 *Changes in self-image and self-esteem*
   Participants reported increased levels of confidence, a fresh perspective on life with aphasia and shifts in their own attitude to disability:

   'It made me think of what I am and why.'

   'You've got to be what you have to be and ... um ... use all the things that are put to you by your ... um ... dis ... what's the word? ... Dis ... disabili ...'

2 *Changes in personal skills and resources*
   Although communication skill work had not been an explicit focus of the group, participants commented on distinct changes in their

communication abilities. These appeared to relate to higher levels of confidence:

'because I've got more confident ... and the words are coming easier to me.'

Group members also noted changes in assertiveness skills and in the management of anger, frustration and anxiety. This contributed for some to a feeling of increased control and autonomy and new patterns of motivation and decision making:

'the self-advocacy class I think is great ... it does um ... wake you up and get you going.'

3 *Changes in interactions and relationships*
Changed skills noted above, in turn had a knock-on effect to communication with and reaction to others. Post course, participants reflected that they were more explicit and assertive about their needs, more robust to the reactions of others and noted improvements in the quality of personal and social relationships:

'Once I've told them (about stroke) they'll walk away or they will come to me.'

Some respondents reported decreased anxiety talking to strangers and greater confidence in dealing with doctors:

I: So a neighbour rang the bell?
R: Yeah ... yeah
I: And you opened the door?
R: Yeah ... yeah
I: And again is that something you would have done before anyway?
R: No ... no ... no

4 *Increased participation in life*
Changes in this area related to an enhanced sense of belonging, going out more and finding new friends. Some participants remarked on a new awareness of the personal, social and political

impact of aphasia and disability and an increased understanding of self-advocacy. Others expressed their desire to participate in an on going self-help group:

'It enables me to find out about other people – they have their stroke victims er experience and the subsequent years and they can pool it.'

The in-depth interviews also revealed group participants' thoughts about the limitations of the group. There was a general feeling that perhaps the best time for such a course was after the acute stage of illness, once major rehabilitation had come to an end (that is, at around two years post onset). Some people felt disappointed that they had not had access to the group earlier. There were strong feelings that the group should have taken place in the morning, not the afternoon. This had fitted the structural needs of the centre, but not the fatigue timetables of participants. Some participants felt that the course was simply too short. By Week 10 they were just reaching a starting point. Sometimes the minutes were too wordy and inaccessible, and more information was required before the course began.

Attribution of change

As an evaluation tool, in-depth interviewing had the added advantage of allowing us to probe participants' ideas regarding the attribution of changes made. Unsurprisingly, some changes were ascribed to the presence of other group members: their ideas, insights, knowledge and shared experience. In common with many other social, therapy or self-help groups, participants reported enjoying and benefiting from the whole group process with its relaxed, supportive atmosphere, opportunity to listen and feel listened to, motivating environment and conversational support:

'The group is very good to listening and speaking.'

However, a number of changes were specifically attributed to the group style, content and focus upon self-advocacy. The features about the group that were valued included:

• The opportunity to reflect on one's whole life

- The opportunity to be more open regarding personal issues
- Discussion of social issues and needs (for example, benefits, discrimination)
- Conversation opportunities as opposed to speech practice
- The differentiation of this group from the more overtly social function of other self-help and conversation groups that some participants had attended
- The portfolio and biography work
- The feeling of being in control of the group's agenda

Celebrating aphasia

In this final section exploring the development of new identities we look at the role of the arts and disability culture in supporting personal growth and self-knowledge. Art, music, dance, mime and creative writing have long been recognised for their potential in promoting healing and personal development. The arts represent, for many people, an important form of recreation, and an integral part of their educational, social and cultural life. The onset of aphasia and mobility difficulties can often severely constrain the opportunities for ongoing participation in and enjoyment of cultural activities, further heightening the sense of exclusion.

Music, images and movement offer a means of expression and communication that can support or circumvent the difficulties posed by compromised language. Drama and music therapies have proved useful in work with children who have severe and profound learning difficulties (Grove & Park, 1996). Art therapy has the potential to enable a client with mental illness or severe language or cognitive impairment to explore otherwise inaccessible internal worlds. A number of mainstream rehabilitation units now employ art therapists. Even in primary health care, there is growing interest in the potential of creative writing for supporting those who wish to explore and express their symptoms and illnesses. For example, some general practice health-care surgeries have established residencies for writers, and some invite patients to keep therapeutic diaries, which can function in lieu of conventional medicine (Bolton, 1998).

Participation in the creative arts not only supports the principles of social inclusion and access but offers an alternative to the powerful medical model paradigm with its focus on impairment, pathology and restitution. Acknowledgement, enjoyment and celebration of difference are ideas that seem fundamentally at odds with traditional medical and rehabilitation thinking. The competence and the uniqueness of the individual is a central theme here, and one which is very influential in the approach to therapy adopted at the aphasia centre.

Clearly, reading or writing poetry, discussing fine art or deconstructing passages of writing are activities that pose interesting challenges to the client–therapist partnership, particularly when language is compromised. We do not underestimate the nature of these challenges, but know from work in other fields that they need not be overwhelming. For example, children with profound learning difficulties have successfully taken part in workshops on *Macbeth* (Grove, 1998) and elderly people with dementia join and enjoy creative writing classes (Killick, 1998). Hopefully some of the ideas we are trying out at the centre (themselves borrowed from other areas of work with people who have language impairments) will strengthen the case for involving and including people with aphasia in literature and the arts.

Many of the activities we describe here are in a developmental stage. They will benefit from creative and analytical thinking around theoretical frameworks and presentation methods, and systematic monitoring of outcome. However, our own experiences thus far, together with the growing body of experiment, enterprise and debate in other areas of health and medicine suggest that this is an area that has great scope for people with aphasia.

Words, pictures and music

Visual imagery

Many therapists will be familiar with visual techniques for enabling clients to communicate past and present experiences. Timelines, representing birth to the present time or the period of recovery since the onset of disability, can be a useful first step to locating the current self in the context of what has gone before and aspirations for the future. Photographs that relate to particular phases or life events are also a concrete way of beginning an exploration, with individuals or groups, of the diverse lives and experiences that impaired language might otherwise render indescribable. Photographs and timelines in this context act as a resource or ramp to support conversation about experience and change. Similarly, discussion about emotions and events can be usefully supported by the wealth of materials in the Pictographic Communication Resources Manual (Kagan *et al*, 1996). Symbols and visual materials can support a client in telling stories that are dynamic and rich in event, emotion and drama, rather than simply the bare bones of fact.

Further opportunities for exploring the inner experience are offered in the endless range of visual material provided by the greetings card industry – a rich source of easily accessible imagery. We use a range of photographs, cartoons, landscapes, abstract, impressionist, romantic, classical and modern art images when working with our clients to help them find a point of reference for their inner state. Such activities support expression of feelings, experiences and dreams where words may not be available or adequate to the complexity of the task. So, for example, asked to focus on how they felt at the time of their stroke, a group of individuals selected images as diverse as Munch's 'The Scream', a bleak black and white Ansel Adams landscape, and a colourful but chaotic abstract by Matisse.

These images gave rise to some illustrative words and phrases, but also provided an interesting visual forum for group members to question, affirm or contrast their own experience with that of others who had faced a similar life-changing event. Selection and discussion of personal issues with the support of such images have enabled groups to address experiences and events relating to hospital, recovery, relationships, and expectations of the future. Unsupported by these images, their narrative may have been less clear or elaborated. Using this method, those with very severely impaired expressive language have some means of participating in a group on equal terms.

Picture selection and representation can also be used as a means of gauging change over time. We have found that one of the most popular and effective ways of measuring subjective experiences of change during attendance at the centre has been the diagram of the 'tree of life' (*see* Figure 5.6).

Clients and caregivers are asked at the beginning of a period of therapeutic input to look at the image and identify where they would locate

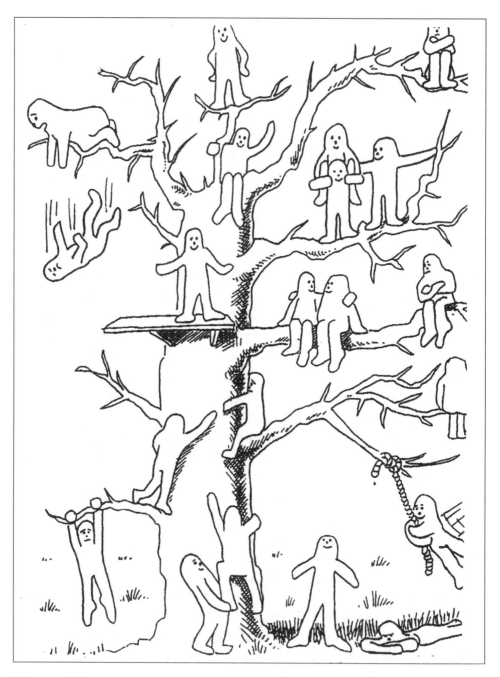

Figure 5.6 The 'tree of life' diagram. (Reproduced from Games Without Frontiers with kind permission of Harper Collins)

themselves within it. They can do this in relation to a number of different factors – for example, how they feel about their level of communication, how confident they feel about being in the group, and the character in the picture who most relates to their current sense of participation. For example, clients may select the isolated character enviously eyeing others on the tree, the harmonious couple or the figure tentatively clinging to the trunk of the tree and reaching up for support. Revisiting the same picture at the end of therapy can enable the client to indicate in a visual and concrete manner subjective changes that might not otherwise have been articulated and that the therapist might have been unable to guess.

The usefulness of diagrams such as these, and the art and photographic images already mentioned is that they take on a different significance for different people, allowing the expression of uniquely individual experience. Therapist and client can use such materials not only to stimulate language but to explore, challenge and learn from a dynamic, three-dimensional interaction of communication, experience and identity. For some clients at the centre, visual art has become a means both of emotional expression and of supporting conversation and connection with others, an enriching experience for everyone concerned.

Music

Many clients at the aphasia centre continue to enjoy music as a recreational activity that has perhaps been less affected by change in language function than some other activities. However, it can also function as a tool to access past experiences and events. Pieces of music can, like the visual images in the preceding section, provide a support for expressing moods, emotions and experiences. At the centre recently, group members selected a piece of music that represented a particular time of their lives, and this led to discussion of personality, preference and lifestyle. Similarly we have run 'Desert Island Discs' sessions in which groups of clients have presented a number of pieces of music representing different moods, phases and events in their lives, both before and after the onset of their communication and other disabilities.

As with visual imagery, the music becomes a support for accessing and using language. Thus, a group at the centre engaged in generating synonyms and language to describe a Mahler symphony and a piece of modern jazz, then used these to communicate subjective states and opinions. However, music can also correct the over focus on the decoding of language as the prime means of receptive communication. Focusing on inference and affective response, the attention shifts away from the impairment and pathology.

Creative writing

The number of autobiographies inspired by illness bears witness to the power of creative writing as a form of cathartic healing and exploration of self. Recent additions to autobiographical accounts of stroke included Jean Dominique Bauby's (1997) striking description of being locked inside paralysis following a brainstem stroke and Robert McCrum's experience of a right-hemisphere stroke (1998). For both authors, writing is a way of finding sense in a time of trauma and change. McCrum writes:

> I began the story with a question, Who am I?, which I have attempted to answer, in my own way, through the stories that make up this narrative. As I have shown, a stroke will open up an almost unending vista of questions about yourself, and your significance. (McCrum, 1998, p215)

Few of the clients whom we meet in therapy have the literary background or preserved language abilities of these eminent authors but, with support, people with aphasia can be encouraged to use creative writing to explore their own landscapes.

Again the therapist is faced with the challenge of access to and expression within a verbal medium that is the very location of the primary impairment. Discussing writing workshops with adults who have learning disabilities, Hunt & Sampson (1998) warn of the need to:

> ensure that both process and product work a balance between prioritising the clients' own way of writing their experiences and the new opportunities and skills which the facilitator can contribute. (Hunt & Sampson, 1998, p13)

What might this mean in the context of aphasia? Therapists can contribute by providing supports for lexical selection and syntactic frameworks. They may resource the session with models from poets and writers and other individuals with aphasia and other impairments who have written about their own experiences. They may facilitate and support the discussion around a piece of writing, or act as scribe in recording the thoughts and sentiments that clients produce in response to materials, personal writings and each other. They may summarise and clarify. They may also support individuals and the group in identifying these creative tracts as, in the words of Ted Hughes (1994), a 'separate literature'. Thus, rather than the aphasic person's language being automatically perceived as flawed or incorrect, the facilitators and poets can help to point out the value, literary uniqueness, power and beauty of the work. These functions are evident in the poetry and aphasia workshops outlined below.

Autobiographical writing that relates to different phases of the past, of the illness and of subsequent recovery sits well within personal portfolio work. People with limited writing ability can use their words or their creative, perhaps scribed, 'voice', to illuminate a series of photographs and memorabilia relating to these periods and events. Individuals who have more facility with written language might integrate creative writing with specific impairment-based goals such as monitoring of verb-argument structures or the use of spell-check and thesaurus strategies in producing material. Photographs of important life events such as births, marriages and holidays might resource creative-writing sessions in which the client is encouraged to recall and write about not just the people and the events, but the sounds, the smells, the colours and the textures of their personal experience.

We have found that some clients enjoy working together to read and discuss extracts from published books and papers. These have the potential to model and stimulate creative writing, especially when they deal with powerful themes such as illness, struggle, loss, achievement, exclusion, discrimination, catharsis and change. In this context, it is worth pointing out that such sessions are geared towards the enjoyment of language and literature, rather than language as the focus of trauma and pathology. Useful texts include:

J-D Bauby (1997): *The Diving-Bell and Butterfly*
R McCrum (1998): *My Year Off*
L Keith (ed)(1994): *Mustn't Grumble*
G Edelman & R Greenwood (eds) (1992): *Jumbly Words*
C Ireland & M Black (1992): *Living with aphasia: the insight story*
Parr *et al* (1997): *Living with Aphasia*

For more extensive discussion of the themes and therapeutic uses of creative writing readers should consult the work of Gillie Bolton (Bolton, 1999).

Celebrating the language of aphasia

LANGUAGE is a gift
LANGUAGE is flowing
LANGUAGE is so powerful
More powerful than before
More scared – more fearful
More demanding – more exhausting
More screamful – more scheming
Not so available and not so understand
(Ireland, 1998a)

Recently at the centre, we have begun to explore aphasia poetry as a means of developing confidence, strength and enjoyment of the new way that people experience language after stroke and brain injury. Much of this work has been inspired by the aphasia poetry of Chris Ireland, a teacher, counsellor and writer who had a stroke 10 years ago leaving her with aphasia and a range of other long-term impairments. She writes:

Living with aphasia is facing daily struggle – pain, confusions, isolating, anxiety – and learning and understanding within the social world – so noisy, so dirty polluted, needy, greedy. (Foreword to *Talking about Aphasia*, Parr *et al*, 1997, pix)

While she never denies the discomforts and complexities of her personal impairments, restrictions imposed by society and her own vulnerability and fragility, Chris has relocated her previous love of language and teaching and channelled it into exploring personal and collective ways of celebrating the language of aphasia:

> In feedback and empowering people to tell their stories, to filter, open hole the stony wall, graphical, strongly, powerful. (Parr *et al*, 1997, pix)

Since 1998 she has been the Poet in Residence at the centre, presenting her work in therapy groups, at poetry workshops and at other events. Her presentations offer some significant challenges to people with receptive language difficulties, to people who have reduced confidence in their ability to be creative and have fun with language and to people who may place a premium on 'correct' language rather than non-standard spellings, pronunciations, word forms and syntax.

Through her experimental performances, Chris has exposed the difficulties inherent in facilitation. Thus, while multimedia devices such as video and music may help create moods and support her poems, they also risk overwhelming some of the audience. Drawings and photographic images help some clients locate key themes of a written poem but have the drawback for some people of being overly concrete and possibly distracting. Some clients have reported finding aphasic language with its 'errors' and inventions as more difficult to follow than standard English.

Chris's work also exposes deep-seated attitudes towards disability, sometimes a raw experience. For some, the language of aphasia poetry is a bright beacon of creativity. They revisit poems such as Lewis Carrol's *Jabberwocky* and claim nonsense verse as a language of their own. Others reject Chris's work totally, regarding it as unfinished, naive and error-laden. Whatever the reaction, however, such sessions have undoubted therapeutic potential in exploring language, standard forms, opinions, experience and difference.

As Chris describes in the poetry extract below, her aphasia is a form of poetry in motion, with a voice and a significance that transcends more traditional, narrow constructions of aphasia as mere language impairment. Chris's broken sentences, fragmented syntax and unusual word associations derive from her aphasia but have a density and originality which is genuinely poetic.

ASPHASIA POETRY IN MOTION
Unavailable by demand!!
Too many words in the world.
WORD – WORLD – WORDY – WORLD !!
We own our words and
Pictures for our new world.

Asphasia – asps – asphasia
Own – our – own personal internal
rhythm.
Labyrinth spirals to the soul.
In motion – pictures – MUSIC – movement
Touch – smell – feel so deeply.
Alive if 'LISTEN TO' !!!

As student and teacher
To share and to understood
TOGETHER
Build up
Compassion , caring world
Lost world and explore word/world and
With asphasia poetry in motion
TO NEW WORD- WORLD !!
(Ireland, 1998b)

Case Study 5.4 The Poetry and Aphasia Group

The experimental poetry and aphasia group ran over a 10-week period. Seven people with mild to moderate aphasia took part. They had been attending the therapy groups at the centre for between three months and almost three years. Participants came from a wide range of social, cultural and occupational backgrounds. One 40-year-old group member, with a pre-stroke passion for poetry and reading, reported she had not gone near her poetry books in the two years since her stroke. Another participant, previously a journalist and actor, had a passion for Shakespeare but had experienced only one rather disappointing visit to the theatre since his stroke. Another person had no previous experience of formal poetry but was a regular church-goer and had greatly enjoyed reading aloud prayers and psalms before her stroke. Another member, a former accountant, reported that he had been put off poetry at school 40 years previously.

Poetry and aphasia were democratically selected as a theme for therapy. The aims of the group were identified as the following:

- To provide group members with opportunities for practising conversational skills and goals
- To develop group members' confidence in expressing opinions
- To enable group members to experiment with new or reconnect with former aspects of recreational activity
- To identify and dismantle barriers to accessing literature in the context of aphasia

The two facilitators, student speech and language therapists, worked with group members to identify personal goals that linked in to these key themes. For example, individual group members selected and presented a poem, song, psalm, or piece of prose to the group, utilising any communication strategies and supports that were current to their therapy. Targets regarding expression of opinions and effective responses to poems were stated and monitored and sessions were videoed to record the nature and dynamics of individuals' inputs to the sessions.

The weekly sessions were varied and diverse. Initially, sessions were framed around pre-prepared materials. For example, a selection of famous poems exploring themes of hope, loss, and love were enlarged and photocopied. Poems on the theme of disability and aphasia were presented in a similar way, discussed, and used as a basis for developing drawings and images of personal experience. Group members were amused and fascinated by a poetry presentation in which singing and rhythm were explored as a way of decoding meaning (see Grove, 1998) and visual materials in the form of fuzzy-felt characters were used to support the telling of the tale of Lord Randall.

As time went on, work became more orientated towards the selections and interests of the group members. So, for example, the Shakespeare admirer hired a video of *As You Like It* and presented a sonnet to music from the film. This led to discussion of ways in which video images, film sequences and the opportunity to replay sections of a film can support understanding where the cut and thrust of live theatre can pose problems. One client talked about a reggae song. A typically quiet member of the group, she demonstrated pride and confidence in her non-standard language as she explained to the group the meaning of the words and led a discussion on variations in culture and language background. Another group member practised hard at reading aloud her favourite Wendy Cope poem before presenting it to the group. Not only did her performance win great applause and laughter from the group, but it represented for her the first reconnection with poetry and her pre-stroke literary identity. The person who had little previous interest in poetry chose to present a piece of illustrated prose from one of his favourite gardening books. The course ended with the production of a group poem, in which visual personal experiences were crafted by the group into a piece about Christmas, using props, synonyms, word associations – all scribed by the facilitators. Participants evaluated this experimental group very positively.

In this chapter, we have started to address the complex issue of aphasia and identity, and have outlined some of the tentative and exploratory therapies that we are using in this area. Clearly, there is scope for further development, both of these approaches and of more sensitive and viable means of evaluating their effects. Therapy that focuses upon identity may seem novel and quite distinct from more familiar therapeutic endeavours, such as supporting communication, or from the very practical work involved in dismantling barriers. Yet it is possible to offer an integrated package of therapy that addresses a number of different issues simultaneously. In the final chapter of this book, we discuss some of the practical aspects, the perils and pitfalls of delivering this kind of service.

CHAPTER 6

Aphasia and Beyond: Real-life Therapy

Introduction

In this final chapter, we give an overview of the therapies for living with aphasia that are continuing to develop and evolve at the aphasia centre, and which have been the subject of this book. We suggest ways in which such a therapy service might be made flexible and responsive to peoples' changing priorities and concerns, given the realities of living with aphasia. Turning to outcomes measurement, we suggest some ways in which therapies might be evaluated. Drawing upon the experience of aphasia therapists working in different settings within the UK, we describe ways in which therapies for living with aphasia might be implemented within different contexts. Finally, we ask in what ways therapies for living with aphasia may be different from more traditional forms of intervention.

What happens in real life?

In this book, we have described a range of therapies for people who are living with long-term aphasia. Clients at the aphasia centre can work individually or in groups and become involved in an ongoing process of negotiation and collaboration. The person with aphasia has the opportunity in therapy both to focus upon the impairment and to tackle some of the long-term issues that arise from it. Work on the use of Total Communication and the training of conversation partners form the basis for developing core communication skills. These skills are the foundation for all the other therapies which we offer including those which seek to dismantle barriers and those which address changes in identity. In this work, the person with aphasia is the central, but not the sole, focus. Caregivers, relatives and other interactants are encouraged and supported in developing their own communication skills, but the scope of therapy also incorporates issues such as rights, access to services and information, and legislation. The overall aim of these interventions is to promote healthy living with aphasia together with choice and autonomy.

In Chapter 1, we described a framework of therapy (Byng *et al*, in press) which incorporates these features. Byng *et al* make the point that such a framework, while clarifying the scope and nature of interventions, somewhat misrepresents a reality that is usually far from neat and orderly. Aphasia therapists will be only too aware that a person's progress through aphasia is rarely a tidy and predictable process. Despite the pressure from resource-managers to do so, it is virtually impossible to foretell the different stages through which an individual will pass, the idiosyncratic interpretations of aphasia and what it means, and the types and durations of therapy which could be useful at different times.

Numerous factors beyond the actual impairment influence the process of learning to live with aphasia. These include the person's emotional state, personality, beliefs regarding the nature and cause of the impairment and how matters might be improved, fears and hopes for the future, and crises and conflicts of identity. All these are experienced in the context of unfolding family dynamics, troubles and celebrations, and the ongoing social, financial and structural difficulties which often accompany long-term impairment. As Elman (1998) points out, such issues profoundly affect both the formulation of goals and the array of therapies on offer.

The key point here, and one reinforced in countless stories and narratives given by people with aphasia (Parr *et al*, 1997), is that adapting to aphasia is not something that occurs in a straightforward, linear fashion. Reaching an understanding of aphasia and integrating it into one's life is often a painfully negotiated and protracted process. Frank (1995) uses the metaphor of travel to capture the experience of illness and disability. The individual does not always 'move forward' at a steady pace and in a straight line, but will at times seem to be changing direction, turning back, spinning into currents, or even immobilised.

Given this somewhat erratic course, the therapist has the potential to become something of a navigator, sensitive to the client's changing position and general direction, aware of the distance already covered and the waters ahead. This may assist the person with aphasia in finding a position, getting bearings and steering a course through sometimes hostile and changing conditions. The process of navigation is conducted through language and communication, through listening, verifying, discussing, checking out and summarising – functions that are often compromised by aphasia and therefore need to be supported. Working with clients, therapists at the centre find themselves continuously revisiting decisions made, going over information, revising and re-stating points reached in previous sessions. While this may, at one level, seem both laborious and time-consuming, its importance in terms of 'navigation' should not be underestimated.

Finding a way through aphasia: different people, different routes

To illustrate the idiosyncratic ways in which people work through aphasia, we are going to describe the routes followed by two clients at the centre. Two vignettes convey the need for therapy to address the inter-relatedness and inter-dependency of the goals of intervention, and changes in these over time, to achieve the overall aim of healthy living with aphasia.

Case Study 6.1 Sonia's story

Sonia is 55 years old and was born in the Dominican Republic, where several members of her extended family still live. She has been resident in the UK for the past 40 years. She is divorced, with three adult children, one of whom lives with her at home. She has a long history of insulin-controlled diabetes. Prior to her stroke, Sonia worked as a care assistant in a local hospital. Her family describe her

245

as having been a very sociable, caring person who was active in her church community. Two years before she came to the centre, Sonia had a series of strokes. These resulted in moderate aphasia, and an exacerbation of pre-existing visual problems. Following her stroke, Sonia became withdrawn and socially isolated. She felt inadequate at church, partly because she felt she could no longer participate in prayer reading and hymn singing. She relied upon her daughter to manage correspondence, financial affairs and household matters.

She had received some local, non-intensive speech and language therapy. This had largely focused on her impairment, particularly targeting her spoken output and her use of practical communication strategies with family and friends. On arrival at the centre Sonia identified her concerns as not being able to talk to people, not being able to read the Bible and finding her new life 'difficult and lonely'. Within the group setting and at coffee sessions she appeared very shy, happy to listen to others but reluctant to initiate any conversation or enter into communication with others unless asked for a response.

Sonia came to the centre over a period of 18 months, attending for two days a week for group and individual therapy. Key themes of group and individual therapy are outlined below and in Table 6.1.

1 *Group sessions*
- Developing an aphasia-friendly leaflet about the centre
- Training conversation partners
- Accessing adult education
- Assertiveness and aphasia
- Health issues
- Poetry and aphasia
- Personal portfolio

2 *Individual sessions*
- Explaining aphasia to family, church friends
- Accessing an advocate
- Semantic comprehension exercises of Bible passages and practising reading aloud

Table 6.1 A framework for interventions – Sonia

Enhancing communication	Identifying and dismantling barriers to social participation	Adaptation of identity	Promoting autonomy and choice	Promoting a healthy psychological state	Health promotion/ Illness prevention
Reading activities: semantic comprehension; key word reading; reading-aloud strategies	Keyworker support in accessing advocate	Learning to participate at church in different way: eg, reading aloud prayers and psalms using strategies	Developing confidence in expressing thoughts and opinions: assertiveness and aphasia, poetry and aphasia	Group discussions re living with aphasia, changes, needs	Accessible information about stroke, aphasia, diabetes, visual impairments in portfolio
Letter writing: developing reference lists for spelling names of relatives; using frameworks to guide ideas and organisation	Developing strategies for accessing information from hospital visits	Reaffirming self with attention to past, present and future: portfolio group sections on family, West Indies, church, interests	Exploring new interests selected by Sonia, eg, exercise class	Expressing emotions, opinions re life, pleasures, losses, hopes, etc – poetry and aphasia	Health issues group: information on risk factors for stroke, healthy living
Portfolio work: developing written reference to explain communication needs to others	Making information accessible, identifying manageable style and presentation of new information	Revealing self to others: presentation of favourite psalm; poetry and aphasia group	Use of portfolio to support and educate others in how to include Sonia in decision making	Accessing new and former interests/roles eg, church activities, exercise class	Stress management

Table 6.1 *Continued*

Enhancing communication	Identifying and dismantling barriers to social participation	Adaptation of identity	Promoting autonomy and choice	Promoting a healthy psychological state	Health promotion/ Illness prevention
Understanding aphasia and its impact on conversations; developing aphasia-friendly leaflet about the centre	Keyworker support in exploring and accessing adult education class which accommodates aphasic needs	Asserting needs and help required from others; understanding aphasia, implications of writing impairments re help with forms and bills	Developing communication strategies to support confidence in difficult situations, eg, talking to builder, doctor	Maintaining connections to church and family based on supported written and spoken communication	Managing encounters with doctors: assertiveness & aphasia group
Training conversation partners group: identifying good/bad partners					

- Strategies to facilitate Bible reading in church
- Developing categorised frameworks to support writing short, social letters to relatives abroad
- Supported portfolio work re stroke and diabetes
- Accessing an exercise class.

Outcomes of therapy for Sonia related to the following areas:

- Specific goal attainment – for example, explaining aphasia to family members, reading aloud of prayers in church with 80 per cent accuracy
- Observed changes in group behaviours – for example, spontaneous initiation of turns, increased mean length of utterance, demonstration of assertive behaviours
- Improved self-rating on scales of confidence in communicative situations
- Improved ratings by peers and therapists on confidence in communication situations at the centre
- Initiation of the decision to leave therapy, having successfully started a twice-weekly exercise class

Case Study 6.2 Sam and June's story

Sam is 59 years old, and prior to his stroke was a lorry driver. He had a left-hemisphere stroke four years before he came to the centre, which left him with a dense right hemiplegia, epilepsy and severe aphasia. He lives with his wife, June, and has four adult children, two of whom live locally. They bring his grandchildren to visit him. Sam is a lifelong Arsenal Football Club supporter.

Sam came to the centre two years ago as a participant on a drawing therapy project for people with severe aphasia. At this time his spoken output was severely impaired, characterised by several social phrases, inconsistent use of 'yes' and 'no' and several recurrent utterances. He made no spontaneous use of drawing or gesture. Sam's comprehension enabled him to take part in everyday conversation, although he had difficulty following longer or more complex material and group discussion.

Socially, Sam appeared withdrawn and uncomfortable communicating with anyone other than June. He was frequently tearful. June reported feeling tired and depressed by her onerous caregiving duties. She had given up her full-time job to be with Sam and felt isolated and saddened by the loss of her former life and no longer spending time with her family and friends.

Sam had attended weekly out-patient therapy at his local hospital for approximately one year. Both Sam and June indicated that they were grateful for this contact, although they felt there had been little change in his communication in recent months. Sam came to the centre for one two-hour session per week while he was taking part in the drawing project. Since then, he has attended two days per week, although he has had frequent periods of ill health during this time. In addition to regular informal involvement with Sam's therapy, June attended a six-week support group for caregivers and brought her daughter along to an information day and to a training for conversation partners.

Key themes of Sam's package of therapy are outlined below, and in Table 6.2.

1 *Group sessions*
- Drawing therapy
- Using Total Communication in everyday environments
- Accessing everyday environments (pub outing project)
- Developing a leaflet to educate relatives about aphasia
- Stress management and aphasia for people with aphasia and their relatives/caregivers
- Developing a video about aphasia

2 *Individual sessions*
- Drawing therapy
- Interaction analysis with Sam and June
- Exploring key word reading
- Developing a personalised communication book
- Semantic categorisation work linked to use of communication book
- Individual counselling sessions

Table 6.2 *A framework for interventions – Sam*

Enhancing communication	Identifying and dismantling barriers to social participation	Adaptation of identity	Promoting a healthy psychological state	Promoting autonomy and choice	Health promotion/ Illness prevention
Total Communication work: drawing therapy, using gesture	Total Communication in everyday environments: physical and communicative barriers to going to pub, museum	Carers group to enable wife to develop own identity and disentangle own from stroke 'victim' perception of husband	Education and support for wife re nature of aphasia, stroke	Use of supported conversation techniques in group and with wife to encourage and enable communicative Sam to participate in decisions	Coping with stress group: understanding physical, emotional, effects of stress
Developing and utilising personalised communication book	Identifying aphasia-friendly formats for leaflets/information materials	Enhanced communication and confidence enables greater participation in family life, role as joker, supporter in group	Individual counselling sessions	Reinforcing notion of competence in education sessions with group and sessions with relatives	Understanding stroke and aphasia: aphasia-friendly information
Training conversation partners leaflet: explaining to others Sam's needs and preferences from conversation partners	Identifying communicative and attitudinal barriers to participation in conversation	Expressing opinions in conversation	Group sessions re aphasia and emotions: use of pictorial materials to support expression of emotional state	Support and education for wife in carers group re ways of re-establishing balance and involvement in decision making	Relatives support group: encouraging June to prioritise own needs and share caregiving role

Table 6.2 *Continued*

Enhancing communication	Identifying and dismantling barriers to social participation	Adaptation of identity	Promoting autonomy and choice	Promoting a healthy psychological state	Health promotion/ Illness prevention
Video work with Sam and wife re supported conversation	Video and leaflet project allow exploration of way other people disable person with aphasia	Participation in group conversations: eg, discussion of current Arsenal performance	Educating others re competence: eg, video project showing communication skills in given situations	Creating opportunities to give feedback on group/centre initiatives: eg, leaflet about centre, student performance	
Input to family members through information and training days		Communication book used to introduce himself to others			

Outcomes of therapy for Sam related to:

- Increased ease and flexibility of communication between Sam and June
- Marked increase in Sam's confidence in the group and in social situations (now well known as the joker in the group and always quick to support other clients)
- Increased use of Total Communication in the group sessions and in social interactions around the centre and at home – for example, when ordering sandwiches
- Use of interactive drawing in conversations at the centre (although this still requires prompting)
- Spontaneous use of a communication book as a means of discussing himself and his personal identity
- Increased understanding by Sam and his family of the nature of aphasia
- Marked changes in June's general well-being, and lessening of her social isolation

As these vignettes suggest, the course which individuals follow through the therapeutic options that we offer will inevitably be guided by their individual interests, personal priorities and the stage reached in their recovery. Decisions regarding therapy will also be influenced by the choices made by group members. As with any group in which individuals have differing ideas and contrasting priorities, the process of negotiation can be a communicatively challenging experience. The framework for therapy described in the case studies is helpful in making the purpose, focus, potential and limitations of the different therapies clear and explicit. Listening carefully to the concerns and issues raised by individual group members, and reflecting on the choices available, clients and therapists together select therapy options which are currently of greatest relevance. Table 6.3 compares the courses of therapy offered to Sam and Sonia and shows how each of the therapy packages was integrated over time.

The process of charting a course through these therapeutic options will be characterised by the regular discussions between the client and keyworker. Goal-setting is never a straightforward process for client or

Table 6.3 *Sonia and Sam – comparing the course of therapy*

Sonia									
Individual — Assessment	Semantic reading	Bible reading strategies	Accessing adult education	Accessing an advocate	Defining aphasia	Portfolio information on health	Handling hospital appts	Letter writing	Accessing adult ed. class
Group	Stroke and aphasia information; Assertiveness and aphasia		Accessing adult education	Training conversation partners	Aphasia-friendly leaflet	Portfolio group		Poetry and aphasia	Health issues
Sam									
Individual — Drawing	Communication book	Semantic therapy		Personal leaflet re aphasia	Communication book	Interaction therapy		Individual counselling	Communication book
Group — Drawing	Total Communication		Drawing and Total Comm.	Leaflet project	Total Comm. in everyday env. project	Stress management		Video project	Stress man. + relatives
	Relatives group				Relatives info. day		Training rels. as conv partners		

therapist but we have found that maintaining an explicit focus upon what clients are going to do after they leave the centre offers them a useful means of charting their passage through therapy. The initial discussion, in which client and therapist explore pressing concerns offers a first opportunity for both partners to find their bearings and to select suitable group and individual therapies.

Evaluation – challenging outcomes

In Chapter 2 we described in more detail the process of collaborative goal setting and the important role that goal setting can play in reviewing progress made in therapy. Of course ongoing review and evaluation of this kind are vital both in focusing (or concluding therapy) and in justifying to managers and funders the impact that interventions have made. While at the centre we acknowledge how fortunate we are to be free of some of the constraints of NHS management and funding streams, we too are required to monitor and articulate the benefits of therapy to justify funding from grant-awarding charities and research bodies.

There have been welcome developments in outcome measurement recently that reinforce the need to take account of disability, handicap and well-being in addition to impairment (Enderby, 1992). A widening range of tools relates measurement in the domain of communication to more 'functional' everyday activities that are not only meaningful to the individual but will carry weight in the argument for continuing funding from third-party payers and service purchasers. Therapists are increasingly exploring quality-of-life measures as a means of trying to capture change in a person's response to and ability to cope with living with disability. Holland & Thompson (1998) and Garrett (1999) offer comprehensive reviews of evaluation tools for measuring change in different areas of therapy within differing healthcare contexts.

New tools such as the ASHA–FACS (Frattali et al, 1995) or the Ryff quality of life scales (1989) offer interesting opportunities for non-impairment based evaluation. However, we continue to be aware of how many of these measures not only fail to capture the subtleties of change which therapies for living with aphasia may bring about, but fail to incorporate the non-professional, insider perspective on change.

Throughout the text and in the case studies in this chapter, we have attempted to describe some of the tools which make up the package of evaluation materials that we use at the centre. Through our experience in both service delivery and aphasia research, we are, like all aphasia clinicians, constantly aware of the need to deliver practical, responsive and well-articulated therapies that can be measured in valid, reliable and meaningful ways. Mindful of the huge advances in monitoring change which carefully focused goals of therapy and systematic, grounded and flexible assessment tools have brought to aphasia therapy in other areas (for example, Kay et al, 1992) we have struggled to maintain greater clarity and focus in living with aphasia therapies. We grapple on a daily basis with the complexities of measuring and articulating the changes which clients derive from group-based therapies, where heterogeneity and multiple layers of group and individual goals of therapy weave colourful and overlapping tapestries of intervention. On a daily basis we continue to confront the puzzling and unanswered questions of outcome from aphasia therapy (Holland & Thompson, 1998). These questions and challenges, which are summarised in Table 6.4, reaffirm the fact that we are at a preliminary stage of developing frameworks for outcome measurement. As Byng et al, 1998 remind us:

> the challenge for speech and language pathology is to ensure that, within the emerging culture, we can continue to provide interventions and services which are both relevant and accessible to clients, and which result in meaningful outcomes. (Byng et al, 1998, p576)

In the context of these challenges and requirements for further development, a growing trend to incorporate qualitative methods and the 'insider' perspective has helped us incorporate more user-centred evaluation tools within the range of measures we use at the centre. Practical methods of accessing and documenting this information may include the following:

- In-depth interview before, during and after a particular course of therapy

Table 6.4 *Questions and challenges in measuring outcome*

The question	The challenge to outcome measurement
What is the role of the aphasia therapist?	Developing and selecting tools appropriate to the whole scope of aphasia therapy
What are the real-life issues facing people with aphasia and their relatives?	Listening to service users rather than using therapist-determined perceptions of what these issues might be
What measurements are meaningful to those who participate in therapy programmes?	Involving service users in the development of alternative methods of measurement
How can we ascertain which component of a therapy package brings about the most effective change?	Being explicit in articulating the different components of living with aphasia therapies and differentially evaluating these separate components
How can we isolate the effects of treatment from change which could be attributed to external or contextual variables?	Establishing the range of external factors which could be contributing to change, eg, client factors (motivation, health, support levels), service factors (staffing levels, amount and type of intervention) and clinician factors (experience, training, philosophy of practice)
What methodologies best capture change in different areas of therapeutic intervention?	Exploring new qualitative methodologies and ways of combining these with more traditional quantitative methods of measuring healthcare
Who benefits most from different types of intervention?	Describing both clients and their therapies in sufficient depth and detail to contribute to a resource of evidence-based practice
When is the best time for treatment and introducing different types of treatment?	Reporting well controlled longitudinal case studies of individuals and groups of individuals who participate in a range of therapies during the course of their interaction with the speech and language therapist
How long should therapy continue for?	Clearly articulating the role and purpose of the therapy package and individual components within the package as a means of negotiating goals and putting timescales on therapies addressing these goals

- Problem identification, rating of feelings relating to identified problems and feedback on any changes in depth/nature of feelings post therapy (*see* Chapter 2)
- Listening to and recording the way clients construct their personal narrative or journey through long-term disability
- Observation of specific behaviours in identified situations or with identified conversation partners
- Analysis of documents written by, with or about participants in therapy
- Analysis of content/themes (as well as form of communication) that clients discuss during, before and after therapy video recordings
- Recording and reporting on identified behaviours, situations, opportunities within aphasia-friendly diaries
- Focus group interviews with participants after specific group therapy programmes
- Aphasia-friendly rating scales evaluating satisfaction/usefulness of particular components of therapy
- Regular audit of goal achievement and change in problem rating for individuals and the group (*see* Chapter 2)

An expanded and creative approach to outcome measurements can form a cornerstone to measuring that important aspect of therapy concerned with the 'moving on with the unfinished business of life.' (Holland & Thompson, 1998, p262) Clearly this moving on will also entail negotiation of how and when to move on from therapy.

Leaving therapy
Given the long-term nature of our involvement with clients, it is important to take regular stock of progress made, to refocus therapy or re-negotiate the nature and role of therapy. The termly review session in which client and keyworker discuss and agree a prepared report can be another important marker in the course through therapy. This meeting provides an opportunity to evaluate whether goals have been met, are still current or require adjustment. Clients contribute to and ultimately take ownership of the reports about their progress. Documents, such as a report or negotiated guidelines regarding some aspect of communication,

can be written in a form which is accessible to the person it relates to and can offer clients and their families a way of understanding, questioning or retaining information which otherwise might remain vague and intangible. An example of one client's accessible guidelines for using the telephone is provided in Figure 6.1.

The process of regular goal setting, reviewing change, re-directing therapy and looking to current and future needs is, as with all therapy, geared towards addressing the timing of 'discharge'. We are somewhat uncomfortable with this term, as it suggests medicalisation, doctor/therapist-driven decisions, and lack of agency on the part of the client. If possible, we prefer to refer to what is undoubtedly a complex and protracted process as 'leaving therapy'. Unsurprisingly, the point at which therapy ends is known to have a profound impact on many users of health services. Pound (1993) found that people with aphasia rarely felt involved in the decision to end therapy. Her respondents felt that therapy finished too soon and often too abruptly. Some people likened the ending of therapy to the experience of bereavement or redundancy. This accords with comments made by respondents in the study by Parr *et al* (1997) who describe the traumatic experience of being suddenly cut off from therapy without preparation or explanation in terms of being 'dumped' and 'abandoned'.

Long-term therapy inevitably brings the threat of dependency to the relationship between client and therapist. Dependency goes both ways – the client needs the therapist and the therapist needs the client, and neither finds it easy to let go. Aware of this, we have begun to evolve structures and practices which promote partnership and seek to create a culture of critical reflection for both parties. Ideally, it is the client who initiates and manages the ending of therapy, as described in Case Studies 6.1 and 6.2. As a rule, the issue of what will happen in the future, how people will spend their time when not attending the centre, how they can find similar or alternative opportunities for socialisation, recreation and work will be addressed explicitly from the outset and at regular intervals.

The process of setting and reviewing goals that have an explicit focus on lifestyle rather than pure change in language and communication will also be constant during the process of therapy. In some cases, it may be precisely the fact that new therapeutic goals are becoming hard to set which indicates therapy is reaching a natural conclusion. In such

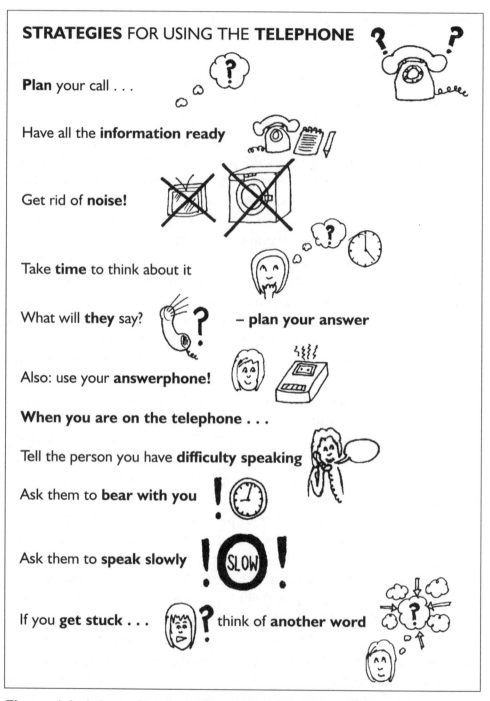

STRATEGIES FOR USING THE **TELEPHONE**

Plan your call . . .

Have all the **information ready**

Get rid of **noise!**

Take **time** to think about it

What will **they** say? – **plan your answer**

Also: use your **answerphone!**

When you are on the telephone . . .

Tell the person you have **difficulty speaking**

Ask them to **bear with you**

Ask them to **speak slowly**

If you **get stuck** . . . think of **another word**

Figure 6.1 *Aphasia-friendly guidelines for using the telephone*

instances, the last phases of therapy might focus explicitly on exploring and accessing socially supportive settings or other communities of aphasic people. Gradually, contact with these communities starts to replace contact with communities based at the centre. This process might include preparation for, visits to and feedback from visits to local self-help or support groups. In some cases, it may also include working with a number of clients over time to support the setting up and/or campaigning for new provision locally.

Leaving therapy should not be rushed. The process of ensuring full involvement, negotiating goals, exploring options, putting in place supports and building confidence and skills to address new ventures and new lifestyles is no easy business and cannot be accomplished quickly. Clients at the centre work towards leaving over a period of at least one 10-week term, but in many cases this process stretches over two to three terms.

The process of leaving therapy thus becomes different from a more service-led therapy package in which it may not be possible to put time into ensuring a collaborative, phased entry into the next stage. Ideally, leaving therapy should highlight new opportunities and the potential for the ongoing development of self-esteem and personal identity, rather than a sudden exit from rehabilitation and a closure to further hope of recovery. Although it can be very hard to face the possibility that their language may not change significantly, many people who start to attend self-help and conversation groups report the continuing development of their confidence and communication skills. Some people return more fully to roles and positions within the family, in work or education. Others enjoy the time and opportunity to participate in new hobbies and interests. By exploring this potential for positive outcomes, we are not, of course, denying the difficulties of living with aphasia and the ongoing struggle which this entails.

'It's all right for you ...': therapies in acute and rehabilitation settings

When we talk to therapists and clinicians about the work of the centre, many point out that their working circumstances and environments are very different from ours. How can therapists working in acute settings or within highly medicalised environments make use of therapies for living with aphasia, particularly when their contact time is limited? These concerns are not just confined to the UK. The advent of managed care in the USA poses a monumental challenge to aphasia therapists concerned with enhancing the quality of life for people with aphasia (Sarno, 1997).

Our setting, and the scope and flexibility of our contracts with clients enable us to address long-term issues with them. However, colleagues within acute and rehabilitation settings have successfully implemented some therapies for living with aphasia, and have started to integrate these within their practice. Their experience suggests that the principles underpinning such therapies are not necessarily at odds with the culture of acute care. In their view, therapists in different settings can address issues such as change in identity, barriers to participation and accessibility, even very early on. This can be done by:

- Creating accessible, aphasia-friendly environments (for example, by ensuring that all notices, posters, and correspondence are clearly expressed, simply laid out, supported with illustrations or pictographs; by ensuring office answerphone messages are slow and clear; by ensuring that staff, such as receptionists, are trained in basic methods of supporting communication).
- Making information accessible to people with aphasia, and modelling this for other disciplines (for example, by bringing aphasia-friendly reports, explanations and guidelines to case conferences and making sure other team members see these; by offering to work with other team members on rendering their information for patients into aphasia-friendly formats; by emphasising the right of the individual to accessible information; by ensuring that any documents employed by the team in user-consultation, such as questionnaires, are accessible).
- Reconfiguring rehabilitation as encompassing adaptation to a new life by starting to address (a) the person's identity and (b) disabling barriers in the environment even in the very early stages of therapy.
- Supporting people with aphasia and relatives at an early stage in being assertive, clear and confident – for example, in accessing benefits and entitlements (by putting on events and open days for relatives and caregivers which give basic information but also offer

guidelines on where and how to access more information and support and how to complain).

- Explicitly acknowledging that conversation partners include relatives, friends, colleagues but also nursing and ward staff, doctors and others, all of whom need training and support from the start (for example, by offering regular, ward-based training sessions in basic communication support techniques; providing training to other staff and volunteers that addresses the social impact of aphasia).

- Modelling user involvement in all decision making and goal planning (for example, by consistently involving clients in decisions about neurosurgery and in case conferences; by providing support and debriefing for clients who wish to participate; by generating accessible minutes of meetings; by organising focus groups of people with aphasia and caregivers as a means of evaluating services).

- Promoting early contact with others who have aphasia, both at a social level and in terms of contact with wider networks.

- Encouraging debate, reflection and awareness concerning attitudes to disability among clients and staff.

- Exploring the challenge of disability theories to rehabilitation process and the identity of rehabilitation workers (for example, by running study days or seminars for staff which raise these issues and offer time for dialogue and debate).

Dilemmas and challenges raised by therapies for living with aphasia

Therapies for living with aphasia are, as yet, embryonic, somewhat tentative and possibly controversial. In this final section, we describe some of the dilemmas and questions which are raised by such therapies, and the challenges which arise, both for the client and for the aphasia therapist. Questions such as these are complex, and the issues are unlikely to be resolved quickly.

We hope that more answers will emerge as practitioners continue to build on the thoughtful, reflective and creative work which has characterised aphasia therapy for decades.

What exactly is the role of the therapist?

With the implementation of the ideas that we have described in this book, the focus falls upon people living with aphasia. The therapist's role may become uncertain for all parties concerned. Is the therapist in fact an advocate? A social worker? A friend? There is a need for all to be clear and explicit about the boundaries and limitations of what is offered. It is equally important, however, for aphasia therapists to be aware of the particular skills and knowledge regarding language and communication that they bring to therapy, and their central role in transferring these skills to others. As the approaches described here may involve a degree of reconfiguration for therapists, it may be useful to set up support networks and to instigate supervision, if possible. This may mean enlisting the support of managers vis-à-vis a new approach, and exploring its potential in terms of cost effectiveness.

If the client is always right, what happens to professional autonomy?

Involving people in all aspects of clinical decision making does not necessarily mean following unquestioningly what a person wants to do in therapy. The aphasia therapist embarks upon a process of listening, clarifying, negotiating, and compromising, but also in developing the ability to be explicit and assertive about their own views.

What happens to the impairment in this form of therapy?

Students who embark upon therapy for living with aphasia often lose sight of the nature and impact of the language impairment and may sometimes feel that it is ultimately irrelevant. However, it should be stressed that such therapies are not a replacement for more traditional impairment-focused work, but should be offered as part of an integrated package. It is not an either/or situation. For many people with aphasia, the impairment is a central concern. The desire for restitution is natural, powerful, and must be acknowledged. Indeed, some individuals may be quite unable to participate in work on barriers and identity until they have a firmer grasp on their language impairment. This is often provided by the process of making it the explicit focus of therapy.

At the centre, we offer specific cognitive neuropsychological therapies which directly address the language impairment and seek to restore or maximise function. However, these are placed within a broad context of other therapies, and the limitations of what each form of therapy can achieve are, as far as possible, made explicit. In addition, therapists' knowledge of linguistic and cognitive impairments directly influences the practice of therapies for living with aphasia. A detailed understanding of the client's language impairment impacts upon:

- The ways in which information is presented
- Methods and strategies for supporting communication
- Specific individual explanations about the nature of the impairment
- How decisions are negotiated, reconfirmed and re-negotiated
- The expectations of clients from session to session regarding the type and timescale of goals set
- The need for repetition and generalisation outside therapy setting
- The type of facilitation used in group and individual interactions
- The integration of impairment-based work within social model projects.

What about the issue of time?

Like the best impairment-focused therapies, therapies for living with aphasia require a structured, detailed, step-by-step approach. They are not quick and easy to implement. The process of service negotiation, preparation of materials, delivery and consolidation make many demands upon therapeutic time – a resource which is often in short supply. The groupwork and individual initiatives described in this book will inevitably demand a creative and flexible approach to the management of time and resources. Therapists wishing to try out some of these ideas may need to make a case for some re-allocation and re-investment of their time, and they may support their case by being clear about the likely outcomes of these therapies. The key issue here is sustainability. Therapies for living with aphasia aim to support people with aphasia in maintaining a sustainable lifestyle, which should ultimately prove to be less demanding of healthcare services.

Haven't we been doing therapy for living with aphasia for years?

Because living with aphasia therapies draw upon and implement traditional therapeutic activities (such as Total Communication) and are concerned with issues which have dogged therapists for decades (such as generalisation), some colleagues hold the view that this approach is nothing new. Indeed, for some it is simply a new version of functional therapy. However, the theoretical foundation is different to that of traditional therapies (Byng *et al*, in press). Therapies for living with aphasia seek to reconfigure existing approaches within changing social, political and healthcare contexts. They draw on recent social movements, post-modernist philosophies and theories that are developing both within and outside the medical culture and which embody a direct challenge to medical assumptions, rituals and traditions. They effectively demand a reappraisal and reconfiguration of the role of the therapist, the nature of 'recovery', the relationship between client and practitioner and the mode of service delivery.

If they are thoughtfully implemented, the activities described here may have the potential to transform the philosophy and practice of aphasia therapy. Ultimately, the therapeutic focus widens to include working on impairment and supporting people with long-term aphasia in maintaining sustainable lifestyles. Taking a different approach to long-held therapeutic traditions does not diminish therapeutic skills and knowledge – rather it makes full use of them. The therapies described in this book are evolving and will continue to develop as different therapists in different settings exert their influence and exercise their creativity. The strength of these therapies lies in the fact that they have evolved in direct response to the thoughts, concerns and feelings expressed by people with long-term aphasia. Learning to listen continues to be the most difficult part of the process.

References

Abberley P, 1991, 'The significance of the OPCS Disability Surveys', Oliver M (ed), *Social work: disabled people and disabling environments*, Jessica Kingsley, London.

Action for Disabled Adults, 1998, *Open Hole the Stony Wall*, ADA, London.

Adair-Ewing SE, 1999, 'Group process, group dynamics and group techniques with neurogenic communication disorders', Elman RJ (ed), *Group treatment of neurogenic communication disorders: the expert clinician's approach*, Butterworth–Heinemann, Boston.

Andersen G, 1997, 'Post-stroke depression and pathological crying: clinical aspects and new pharmacological approaches', *Aphasiology* 11, 7, pp651–65.

Aten JL, Caliguiri MP & Holland AL, 1982, 'The efficacy of functional communication therapy for chronic aphasia patients', *Journal of Speech and Hearing Disorders* 47, pp93–6.

Bardach JC, 1969, 'Group sessions with wives of aphasic patients', *International Journal of Group Psychotherapy* 19, pp361–5.

Barnes C, 1996 'Theories of disability and the origins of the oppression of disabled people in western society', Barton L (ed), *Disability and society: emerging issues and insights*, Longman, London.

Barrow R, 1999, 'The co-construction of aphasia therapy: taking your cue from the person with aphasia', paper presented at IASLT Conference, Dublin.

Bauby J-D, 1997, *The Diving-Bell and Butterfly*, Fourth Estate, London.

Bellaire KJ, Georges JB & Thompson CK, 1991, 'Establishing functional communication board use for non-verbal aphasic subjects', Prescott TE (ed), *Clinical Aphasiology Proceedings, Vol 19*, Pro-Ed, Austin.

Benson DF, 1980, 'Psychiatric problems in aphasia', Sarno MT & Hook O (eds), *Aphasia: assessment and treatment*, Almquist and Wiksell, Stockholm.

Beukelman D & Mirenda P, 1992, *Augmentative and alternative communication: management of severe communication disorders in children and adults*, Paul H. Brookes, Baltimore.

Beukelman D, Yorkston K & Dowden P, 1985, *Communication augmentation: a casebook of clinical management*, College Hill Press, San Diego.

Blackstone S, 1991a, 'Persons with severe aphasia: what does AAC have to offer?', *Augmentative Communication News* 4, 1, pp1–3.

Blackstone S, 1991b, 'When functional communication is the goal', *Augmentative Communication News* 4, 1, pp4–5.

Boazman S, 1999, 'Inside aphasia', Corker M & French S (eds), *Disability discourse*, Open University Press, Buckingham.

Bollinger RL, Musson ND & Holland A, 1993, 'A study of group communication intervention with chronically aphasic persons', *Aphasiology* 7, 3, pp301–13.

Bolton G, 1998, 'Writing or pills? Therapeutic writing in primary health care', Hunt C & Sampson F (eds), *The self on the page*, Jessica Kingsley, London.

Bolton G, 1999, *The therapeutic potential of creative writing*, Jessica Kingsley, London.

Booth S & Perkins L, 1999, 'The use of conversation analysis to guide individualised advice to carers and evaluate change in aphasia: a case study', *Aphasiology* 13, 4/5, pp283–304.

Booth S & Swabey D, 1999, 'Group training in communication skills for carers of adults with aphasia', *International Journal of Language and Communication Disorders* 34, 3, pp291–310.

Booth T, 1996, 'Sounds of still voices: issues in the use of narrative methods with people who have learning difficulties', Barton L (ed), *Disability and society: emerging issues and insights*, Longman, London.

Brumfitt S, 1993, 'Losing your sense of self: what aphasia can do', *Aphasiology* 7, 6, pp569–74.

Brumfitt SM & Sheeran P, 1997, 'An evaluation of short-term therapy for people with aphasia', *Disability and Rehabilitation* 19, 6, pp221–30.

Bury M, 1991, 'The sociology of impairment: a review of research and prospects', *Sociology of Health and Illness* 13, 4, pp451–68.

Byng S, Kay J, Edmundson A & Scott C, 1990, 'Aphasia tests reconsidered', *Aphasiology* 4, 1, pp67–93.

Byng S, Swinburn K & Pound C (eds), 1999, *The Aphasia Therapy File*, Psychology Press, Hove.

Byng S, Pound C & Parr S, in press, 'Living with aphasia: frameworks for therapy interventions', Papathanasiou I (ed), *Acquired neurological communication disorders: a clinical perspective*, Whurr Publishers, London.

Byng S, Van der Gaag A & Parr S, 1998, 'International initiatives in outcomes measurement: a perspective from the United Kingdom', Frattali C (ed), *Measuring outcomes in speech and language pathology*, Thieme, New York.

Clarke H, 1998, 'Harry's story: becoming a counsellor following a stroke', Syder D (ed), *Wanting to talk*, Whurr Publishers, London.

Coelho CA, 1991, 'Manual sign acquisition and use in two aphasic subjects', Prescott TE (ed), *Clinical Aphasiology Proceedings, Vol. 19*, Pro-Ed, Austin.

Coles R & Eales C, 1999, 'The aphasia self-help movement in Britain: a challenge and an opportunity', Elman R (ed), *Group treatment of neurogenic communication disorders*, Butterworth–Heinemann, Boston.

Communications Forum, 1998, *Living with communication impairment*, Communications Forum, London.

Corbett J, 1989, 'The quality of life in the "independence" curriculum', *Disability, Handicap and Society* 4, 2, pp145–63.

Corker M, 1996, *Deaf transitions: images and origins of deaf families, deaf communities and deaf identities*, Jessica Kingsley, London.

Corker M, 1998, *Deaf and disabled or deafness disabled?* Open University Press, Buckingham.

Corker M & French S, 1999, *Disability discourse*, Open University Press, Buckingham.

Coulter A, 1997, 'The pros and cons of shared decision-making', *Journal of Health Services Policy* 2, 2, pp112–21.

Crow L, 1992, 'Renewing the social model of disability', *Coalition, July*, Greater Manchester Coalition of Disabled people.

Cubelli R, 1995, 'More on drawing in aphasia therapy', *Aphasiology* 9, 1, pp78–83.

D'Afflitti JG & Weitz GW, 1974, 'Rehabilitating the stroke patient: patient-family groups', *International Journal of Group Psychotherapy* 25, pp323–32.

Davis GA & Wilcox MJ, 1985, *Adult aphasia rehabilitation: applied pragmatics,* NFER–Nelson, Windsor.

Dewart H & Summers S, 1996, *Pragmatics profile of everyday communication skills in adults,* NFER–Nelson, Windsor.

Devlin S & Canning Y, 1999, *Automatic text simplification for readers with aphasia,* paper presented at the British Aphasiology Society Biennial International Conference, London.

Edelman G & Greenwood R (eds), 1992, *Jumbly words, and rights where wrongs should be,* Far Communications, Kibworth.

Elman RJ, 1998, 'Diversity in aphasiology: let us embrace it', *Aphasiology* 12, 6, pp456–57.

Elman RJ, 1999, 'Introduction to group treatment of neurogenic communication disorders', Elman RJ (ed), *Group treatment of neurogenic communication disorders: the expert clinician's approach,* Butterworth–Heinemann, Boston.

Elman RJ & Bernstein-Ellis E, 1999a, 'The efficacy of group communication treatment in adults with chronic aphasia', *Journal of Speech, Language and Hearing Research* 42, 2, pp411–9.

Elman RJ & Bernstein-Ellis E, 1999b, 'Aphasia group communication treatment: the Aphasia Centre of California approach', Elman RJ (ed), *Group treatment of neurogenic communication disorders: the expert clinician's approach,* Butterworth–Heinemann, Boston.

Elwyn G & Gwyn R, 1999, 'Stories we hear and stories we tell: analysing talk in clinical practice', Greenhalgh T & Hurwitz B (eds), *Narrative based medicine,* BMJ Books, London.

Enderby P, 1992, 'Outcome measures in speech therapy: impairment, disability, handicap and distress', *Health Trends* 24, 2, pp61–4.

Fawcus M, 1989, 'Group therapy: a learning situation', Code C & Muller D (eds) *Aphasia therapy,* Whurr, London.

Fawcus M, 1992, 'Group work with the aphasic adult', Fawcus M (ed*), Group encounters in speech and language therapy,* Far Communications, Kibworth.

Fawcus M, Kerr J, Whitehead S & Williams R, 1990, *Aphasia therapy in practice: expression*, Speechmark Publishing, Bicester.

Finkelstein V, 1991, 'Disability: an administrative challenge (the health and welfare heritage)', Oliver M (ed), *Social work, disabled people and disabling environments*, Jessica Kingsley, London.

Finkelstein V & French S, 1993, 'Towards a psychology of disability', Swain J, Finkelstein V, French S & Oliver M (eds), *Disabling barriers – enabling environments*, Sage, London.

Frank AW, 1995, *The wounded storyteller*, Chicago University Press, Chicago.

Frattali C, Thompson C, Holland A, Wohl C & Ferketic M, 1995, *American Speech-Language-Hearing Association Functional Assessment of Communication Skills for adults*, ASHA, Rockville.

French S, 1993, 'What's so great about independence?', Swain J, Finkelstein V, French S & Oliver M (eds), *Disabling barriers – enabling environments*, Sage, London.

French S, 1994, 'Disabled people and professional practice', French S (ed), *On equal terms: working with disabled people*, Butterworth–Heinemann, Oxford.

Friedman MH, 1961, 'On the nature of repression in aphasia', *Archives of General Psychiatry* 5, pp252–6.

Gainotti G, 1997, 'Emotional, psychological and psychosocial problems of aphasic patients: an introduction', *Aphasiology* 11, 7, pp635–51.

Gainotti G, Silveri MC, Villa G & Caltagirone C, 1983, 'Drawing objects from memory in aphasia', *Brain* 106, pp613–22.

Garrett K, 1999, 'Measuring outcomes of group therapy', Elman RJ (ed), *Group treatment of neurogenic communication disorders: the expert clinician's approach*, Butterworth–Heinmann, Boston.

Garrett K, Beukelman, D & Low-Morrow D, 1989, 'A comprehensive augmentative communication system for an adult with Broca's aphasia', *Augmentative and Alternative Communication*, pp55–61.

Goldsmith M, 1996, *Hearing the voice of people with dementia*, Jessica Kingsley, London.

Goodwin C, 1995, 'Co-constructing meaning in conversations with an aphasic man', Jacoby S & Och E (eds), *Research on language and social interaction (special issue on co-construction)*, pp223–60.

Green G, 1982, 'Assessment and treatment of the adult with severe aphasia: aiming for functional generalization', *Australian Journal Of Human Communication Disorders* 10, pp11–23.

Green G, 1984, 'Communication in aphasia therapy: some of the procedures and issues involved', *British Journal of Disorders of Communication* 19, pp35–46.

Greenhalgh T & Hurwitz B (eds), 1999, *Narrative based medicine*, BMJ Books, London.

Grist E, Mortley J & Easton J, 1993, 'Communication opportunities for global dysphasics', *Human Communication*, August, pp8–10.

Grove N, 1998, *Literature for all*, David Fulton Publishers, London.

Grove N & Park K, 1996, *Odyssey Now*, Jessica Kingsley, London.

Hay WM, Hay LR, Angle HV & Nelson RO, 1979, 'The reliability of problem identification in the behavioural interview', *Behavioural Assessment* VI, pp107–18.

Helm-Estabrooks N & Holland A, 1998, 'The power of one: every aphasia treatment case is a case study', Helm-Estabrooks N & Holland A (eds), *Approaches to the treatment of aphasia*, Singular Publishing Group, San Diego.

Hevey D, 1992, *The creatures time forgot*, Routledge, London.

Hitchings A, 1992, 'Working with adults with a learning disability in a group setting', Fawcus M (ed), *Group encounters in speech and language therapy*. Far Communications, Kibworth.

Hoen B, Thelander M & Worsley J, 1997, 'Improvement in psychological well-being of people with aphasia and their families: evaluation of a community-based programme', *Aphasiology* 11, 7, pp681–91.

Hogan A, 1999, 'Carving out a space to act: acquired impairment and contested identity', Corker M & French S (eds), *Disability discourse*, Open University Press, Buckingham.

Holland AL, 1982, 'Observing functional communication of aphasic adults', *Journal of Speech and Hearing Disorders* 47, pp50–6.

Holland AL, 1991, 'Pragmatic aspects of intervention in aphasia', *Journal of Neurolinguistics* 6, 2, pp197–211.

Holland AL & Beeson PM, 1993, 'Finding a new sense of self: what the clinician can do to help', *Aphasiology* 7, pp569–91.

Holland AL & Beeson PM, 1999, 'Aphasia groups: the Arizona experience', Elman RJ (ed), *Group treatment of neurogenic communication disorders: the expert clinician's approach*, Butterworth–Heinemann, Boston.

Holland A & Thompson C, 1998, 'Outcomes measurement in aphasia', Frattali C (ed), *Measuring outcomes in speech and language pathology*, Thieme, New York.

Holland S & Ward C, 1990, *Assertiveness: a practical approach*, Speechmark Publishing, Bicester.

Horton S, Mudd D & Lane J, 1998, 'Is anyone speaking my language?', *International Journal of Language and Communication Disorders* 33 (Supplement 1998), pp126–31.

Hughes T, 1994, *Winter pollen*, Faber and Faber, London.

Hughes W & Paterson K, 1997, 'The social model of disability and the disappearing body: towards a social model of impairment', *Disability and Society* 12, 3, pp325–40.

Hunt C & Sampson F, 1998, *The self on the page*, Jessica Kingsley, London.

Hux K, Beukelman D & Garrett K, 1994, 'Augmentative and alternative communication for persons with aphasia', Chapey R (ed), *Language intervention strategies in adult aphasia*, 4th edn, Williams & Wilkins, Baltimore.

Ireland C, 1998a, 'Asphasia poetry in motion', unpublished.

Ireland C, 1998b, 'Language rebel', unpublished.

Ireland C & Black M, 1992, 'Living with aphasia: the insight story', *UCL Working Papers in Linguistics* 4, pp355–8.

Ireland C & Wotton G, 1996, 'Time to talk: counselling for people with dysphasia', *Disability and Rehabilitation* 18, 11, pp585–91.

Jeffers S, 1987, *Feel the fear and do it anyway*, Arrow, London.

Jordan L, 1998, 'Diversity in aphasiology: a social science perspective', *Aphasiology* 12, 6, pp474–80.

Jordan L & Kaiser W, 1996, *Aphasia: a social approach*, Chapman Hall, London.

Kagan A, 1995, 'Revealing the competence of aphasic adults through conversation: a challenge to health professionals', *Topics in Stroke Rehabilitation* 2, 1, pp15–28.

Kagan A, 1998, 'Supported conversation for adults with aphasia: methods and resources for training conversation partners', *Aphasiology* 12, 9, pp816–30.

Kagan A & Cohen-Schneider R, 1999, 'Groups in the introductory program at the Pat Arato Aphasia Centre', Elman RJ (ed), *Group treatment of neurogenic communication disorders: the expert clinician's approach*, Butterworth–Heinemann, Boston.

Kagan A & Gailey G, 1993, 'Functional is not enough: training conversation partners for aphasic adults', Holland AL & Forbes MM (eds), *Aphasia treatment: world perspectives*, Chapman & Hall, London.

Kagan A, Winckel J & Schumway E, 1996, *Pictographic Communication Resources Manual*, Aphasia Centre, North York, Toronto.

Kay J, Lesser R & Coltheart M, 1992, *Psycholinguistic Assessment of Language Processing in Aphasia*, Lawrence Erlbaum Associates, London.

Kearns K, 1986, 'Group therapy in aphasia: theoretical and practical considerations', Chapey R (ed), *Language intervention strategies in adult aphasia*, 2nd edn, Williams & Wilkins, Baltimore.

Keith L (ed), 1994, *Mustn't Grumble*, The Women's Press, London.

Killick J, 1998, 'A matter of life and death of the mind: creative writing and dementia sufferers', Hunt C & Sampson F (eds), *The self on the page*, Jessica Kingsley, London.

Kirk A & Kertesz A, 1989, 'Hemispheric contributions to drawing', *Neuropsychologia* 27, pp881–6.

Kleinmann A, 1988, *The illness narratives*, Basic Books, Harvard.

Knight N & McQueen A, 1998, 'Fashionable?' *Dazed and Confused*, September issue.

Kraat AW, 1990, 'Augmentative and alternative communication: does it have a future in aphasia rehabilitation?', *Aphasiology* 4, 4, pp321–38.

Kunin T, 1955, 'The construction of a new type of attitude measure', *Personal Psychology* 8, pp65–78.

Lawson R & Fawcus M, 1999, 'Increasing effective communication using a total communication approach', Byng S, Swinburn K & Pound C (eds), *The Aphasia Therapy File*, Psychology Press, Hove.

Le Dorze G & Brassard C, 1995, 'A description of the consequences of aphasia on aphasic persons and their relatives, based on the WHO model of chronic diseases', *Aphasiology* 9, 3, pp239–55.

Le May M, 1993, 'Group dynamics', *Therapy Weekly*, December.

Leiwo M, 1994, 'Aphasia and communicative speech therapy', *Aphasiology* 8, 5, pp467–82.

Lesser R & Algar L, 1995, 'Towards combining the cognitive neuropsychological and the pragmatic in aphasia therapy', *Neuropsychological Rehabilitation* 5, 1/2, pp67–92.

Lesser R & Milroy L, 1993, *Linguistics and aphasia: psycholinguistic and pragmatic aspects of intervention*, Longman, London.

Levenson R & Farrell C, 1998, *Public health and the PAMS*, King's Fund Institute, London.

Levinson SC, 1983, *Pragmatics*, Cambridge University Press, Cambridge.

Light J, 1988, 'Interaction involving individuals using augmentative and alternative communication systems: state of the art and future directions', *Augmentative and Alternative Communication* 4, 2, pp66–82.

Luterman D, 1991, *Counselling the communicatively disordered and their families*, Pro-Ed, Austin.

Lyon JG, 1995, 'Drawing: its value as a communication aid for adults with aphasia', *Aphasiology* 9, pp33–50.

Lyon JG, Cariski D, Keisler L, Rosenbek J, Levine R, Kumpula J, Ryff C, Coyne S & Levine J, 1997, 'Communication Partners: enhancing participation in life and communication for adults with aphasia in natural settings', *Aphasiology* 11, pp693–708.

Lyon JG & Helm-Estabrooks N, 1987, 'Drawing: its communicative significance for expressively restricted aphasic adults', *Topics in Language Disorders* 8, pp61–71.

Lyon JG & Sims E, 1989, 'Drawing: its use as a communicative aid with aphasic and normal adults', Prescott T (ed), *Clinical Aphasiology Proceedings, Vol 18*, College Hill Press, San Diego.

Maclaren J, 1996, 'Rehabilitation through advocacy and empowerment', *British Journal of Therapy and Rehabilitation* 3, 9, pp492–7.

McCrum R, 1998, *My Year Off*, Picador, London.

Milroy L & Perkins L, 1992, 'Repair strategies in aphasic discourse: towards a collaborative model', *Clinical Linguistics* 6, 1&2, pp27–40.

Mishler E, 1984, *The discourse of medicine: dialectics of medical interviews*, Ablex, New Jersey.

Morris J, 1998, *Still missing? The experience of disabled children and young people living away from their families*, Who Cares? Trust, London.

Mulhall DJ, 1978, *Personal Questionnaire Rapid Scaling Technique*, NFER, Windsor.

Nettleton S, 1995, *The sociology of health and illness*, Blackwell, Cambridge.

Nichols F, Varchevker A & Pring T, 1996, 'Working with people with aphasia and their families: an exploration of the use of family therapy techniques', *Aphasiology* 10, 8, pp767–81.

Nichols K & Jenkinson J, 1991, *Leading a support group*, Chapman Hall, London.

Oliver M, 1996, *Understanding disability: from theory to practice*, Macmillan, London.

Oxenham D, 1994, 'From frogs into princes: transforming our knowledge base into models of communication that are relevant to people in their environment', *Aphasiology* 8, pp488–91.

Parr S & Byng S, in press, 'Perspectives and priorities: accessing user views in functional communication assessment', Worrall L & Frattali C (eds) *Neurogenic communication disorders: a functional approach*, Thieme, New York.

Parr S, Byng S, Gilpin S & Ireland C, 1997, *Talking about aphasia: living with loss of language after stroke*, Open University Press, Buckingham.

Parr S, Pound C, Byng S & Long B, 1999, *The Aphasia Handbook*, Connect Press, London.

Parsloe P & Stevenson O, 1993, *Community care and empowerment*, Joseph Rowntree Foundation, York.

Parsons T, 1967, *The social system*, Routledge and Kegan Paul, London.

Penman T, 1998, 'Self-advocacy and aphasia', *Bulletin of the Royal College of Speech and Language Therapists*, August.

Peters S, 1996, 'The politics of disability identity', Barton L (ed), *Disability and Society: emerging issues and insights*, Longman, London.

Peters, S, 1999, 'Transforming disability identity through critical literacy and the cultural politics of language', Corker M & French S (eds), *Disability discourse*, Open University Press, Buckingham.

Pound C, 1993, 'Attitudes to disability: power and the therapeutic relationship', British Aphasiology Society Conference, Warwick.

Pound C, 1996, 'New approaches to long-term aphasia therapy and support', *Bulletin of the Royal College of Speech and Language Therapists*, August.

Pound C, 1998, 'Power, partnerships and perspectives: social model approaches to long term aphasia therapy and support', paper presented at the 8th International Aphasia Rehabilitation Conference, South Africa.

Pound C & Parr S, 1998, 'Caregiving and coping: evaluating a support group for relatives of people with long term aphasia', paper presented at the 8th International Aphasia Rehabilitation Conference, South Africa.

Pulvermuller F & Roth VM, 1991, 'Communicative aphasia treatment as a further development of PACE therapy', *Aphasiology* 5, pp39–50.

Pyatak Fletcher P, 1997, 'AAC and adults with acquired disabilities', Glennen SL & De Coste DC (eds), *The handbook of augmentative and alternative communication*, Singular Publishing Group, San Diego.

Rao PR, 1994, 'Use of Amer-Ind code by persons with aphasia', Chapey R (ed) *Language Intervention Strategies in Adult Aphasia*, 3rd edn, Williams & Wilkins, Baltimore.

Ricco-Schwartz S, 1982, 'Fostering an empathetic approach: an in-service curriculum for non-medical professionals, para-professionals and families of aphasic clients', *Gerontology and Geriatrics Education* 2, pp199–206.

Rice B, Paull A & Muller D, 1987, 'An evaluation of a social support group for spouses of aphasic partners', *Aphasiology* 1, 3, pp247–56.

Royal College of Speech and Language Therapists (RCSLT), 1996, *Communicating Quality: professional standards for speech and language therapists*, RCSLT, London.

Ryff C, 1989, 'Scales of psychological well-being (short form)', *Journal of Personality and Social Psychology* 57, pp1069–81.

Sacchett C, Byng S, Marshall J & Pound C, 1999, 'Drawing together: evaluation of a therapy programme for severe aphasia', *International Journal of Language and Communication Disorders* 34, 3, pp265–89.

Sacchett C & Lindsay J, 1998, 'Communicative drawing for severe aphasia: revealing competence and rebuilding identity', paper presented at the British Aphasiology Society Therapy Symposium, Madingley, Cambridge.

Sarno MT, 1997, 'Quality of life in aphasia in the first post-stroke year', *Aphasiology* 11, 7, pp665–79.

Schegloff EA, Jefferson G & Sacks H, 1977, 'The preference for self-correction in the organisation of repair in conversation', *Language* 53, 2, pp361–82.

Schiffrin D, 1988, 'Conversation analysis', Neumayer FL (ed) *Linguistics: The Cambridge Survey IV. Language: the sociocultural context*, Cambridge University Press, Cambridge.

Schneider-Corey M & Corey G, 1997, *Groups: process and practice*, Brooks/Cole Publishing Company, Pacific Grove.

Shapiro MB, 1961, 'A method of measuring psychological changes specific to the individual psychiatric patient', *British Journal of Medical Psychology* 34, pp151–5.

Simmons-Mackie N, 1998, 'In support of supported conversation for adults with aphasia', *Aphasiology* 12, 9, pp831–38.

Simmons-Mackie N & Damico J, 1995, 'Communicative competence and aphasia: evidence from compensatory strategies', Lemme M (ed), *Clinical Aphasiology, Vol 23*, Pro-Ed, Austin.

Sontag S, 1978, *Illness as Metaphor*, Vintage, New York.

Syder D (ed), 1998, *Wanting to talk: counselling case studies in communication disorders*, Whurr Publishers, London.

Thelander MJ, Hoen B & Worsley J, 1994, *York-Durham Aphasia Center: report on the evaluation of effectiveness of a community program for adults*, York Durham Aphasia Center, Ontario.

Thomas C, 1999, 'Narrative identity and the disabled self', Corker M & French S (eds), *Disability discourse*, Open University Press, Buckingham.

Thompson CK, 1998, 'Treating sentence production in agrammatic aphasia', Helm-Estabrooks N & Holland A (eds), *Approaches to the treatment of aphasia*, Singular Publishing Group, San Diego.

Trupe EH, 1986, 'Training severely aphasic patients to communicate by drawing', paper presented at the American Speech-Language-Hearing Association Convention, Detroit.

Tyne A, 1994, 'Taking responsibility and giving power', *Disability and Society* 9, 2, pp249–54.

Wahrborg P & Borenstein P, 1988, 'Progressive psychological deterioration in aphasic and non-aphasic stroke patients', Wahrborg P (ed), *After stroke: behavioral changes and therapeutic intervention in* *aphasics and their relatives following stroke,* thesis, University of Gothenburg.

Wahrborg P, Borenstein P, Linell S, Hedburg-Borenstein E & Asking M, 1997, 'Ten year follow-up of young aphasic participants in a 34-week course at a Folk High School', *Aphasiology* 11, 7, pp709–17.

Waller A, Dennis F, Brodie J & Cairns AY, 1998, 'Evaluating the use of TalksBac, a predictive communication device for nonfluent adults with aphasia', *International Journal of Language and Communication Disorders* 33, 1, pp45–70.

Whitaker DS, 1989, *Using groups to help people*, Routledge, London.

Wilkinson R, 1995a, 'Doing "being ordinary": aphasia as a problem of interaction', Kersner M & Peppe S (eds), *Work in progress, Vol 5*, Department of Human Communication Science, University College London, London.

Wilkinson R, 1995b, 'Aphasia: conversation analysis of a non-fluent aphasic person', Perkins M & Howard S (eds), *Case studies in clinical linguistics*, Whurr Publishers Ltd, London.

Wilkinson R, Bryan K, Lock S, Bayley K, Maxim J, Bruce C, Edmundson A & Moir D, 1998, 'Therapy using conversation analysis: helping couples adapt to aphasia in conversation', *International Journal of Language and Communication Disorders* 33 (Supplement 1998), pp144–9.

World Health Organisation, 1980, *International classification of impairments, disabilities and handicaps*, World Health Organisation, Geneva.

World Health Organisation, 1999, *International classification of functioning and disability, Beta-2 draft, full version*, World Health Organisation, Geneva.

Index

INDEX